THE PREGNANCY SOURCEBOOK

Also by M. Sara Rosenthal

The Thyroid Sourcebook (Lowell House, 1993, 1995)

The Gynecological Sourcebook (Lowell House, 1994, 1995)

The Fertility Sourcebook (Lowell House, 1995)

The Breastfeeding Sourcebook (Lowell House, 1995)

The Pregnancy Sourcebook

Everything You Need to Know

M. Sara Rosenthal

Lowell House
Los Angeles

Contemporary Books
Chicago

To my sister

Library of Congress Cataloging-in-Publication Data

Rosenthal, M. Sara.
    The pregnancy sourcebook : everything you need to know / M. Sara Rosenthal.
        p.   cm.
    Includes bibliographical references and index.
    ISBN 1-56565-156-1
    1. Pregnancy. 2. Childbirth. I. Title.
    RG525.R765   1994
    618.2—dc20   94-22872
                                                              CIP

Requests for such permissions should be addressed to:
Lowell House
2029 Century Park East, Suite 3290
Los Angeles, CA 90067

Lowell House books can be purchased at special discounts when ordered in bulk for premiums and special sales. Contact Department VH at the address above.

Publisher: Jack Artenstein
General Manager, Lowell House Adult: Bud Sperry
Text Design: Mary Ballachino/Merrimac Design

Manufactured in the United States of America
10 9 8 7 6 5 4 3 2 1

Acknowledgments

If it weren't for the commitment, hard work, and guidance of the following people, this book would never have been written: Suzanne Pratt, M.D., F.A.C.O.G., in private practice in Rome, Georgia, who served as my medical adviser; my research assistant, Ellen Tulchinsky, B.A., M.L.I.S.; my editorial assistant, journalist Laura Tulchinsky, B.A.; my editor, Bud Sperry; and my copyeditors, Carolyn Wendt and Dianne J. Woo.

Special thanks to the physicians and health practitioners who donated their time and expertise: Gillian Arsenault, M.D., I.B.C.L.C.; Sue Johanson, R.N., sex educator and counselor; Debra Lander, M.D., F.R.C.P. (C.); Matthew Lazar, M.D., F.R.C.P. (C.), F.A.C.P.; Kelly S. MacDonald, M.D., F.R.C.P. (C.); Lori Moore, M.D., F.R.C.P. (C.); Michael Policar, M.D., F.A.C.O.G.; Frank G. Pratt, M.D., F.A.C.P.; and Daniel Rappaport, M.D., F.R.C.P.(C.).

Finally, in the moral support department, special thanks to my husband, Gary S. Karp, and all the relatives and friends who cheered me on.

Contents

Foreword

The last two years have seen advances in the science of human reproduction that would have stretched the imaginations of science fiction writers. Women today have an astounding control over their reproductive destinies through modern contraceptive methods and a proliferation of new techniques in endocrinology and infertility surgery. The potential now exists for the in utero treatment of the fetus, salvage of babies born too soon or too small, and extension of a woman's reproductive lifespan into her seventh decade. Antibiotics, safer anesthesia, and blood transfusion have made pregnancy and childbirth safer for mother and baby. Maternal deaths in the countries of the developed world are now rare, and increasing attention is paid to the second obstetrical patient: the fetus. Fortunately, most pregnancies proceed quite normally with a minimum of technology and intervention.

The Pregnancy Sourcebook will guide you through the miraculous physiological process involved with the creation of a new human life. Here, you will find discussions of what to expect during pregnancy, childbirth, and the period immediately following delivery. There are explanations of common problems during pregnancy, information on prenatal testing, and such issues as indications for cesarean sections, vaginal birth after cesarean (VBAC), and forceps delivery.

There is perhaps no more intimate medical relationship than that between a pregnant woman and the person who delivers her child. Therefore, choose someone with whom you feel comfortable. As the patient, it is your responsibility to provide an accurate and complete medical history of such factors as past abortions, or sexually transmitted diseases. One of the most useful things you can do to help your doctor during any pregnancy is to keep a written record of your menstrual periods.

It is the responsibility of the midwife or physician to be competent and compassionate. He or she will share your joy when pregnancy goes right, and your sorrow when things go wrong. You should never hesitate to ask for more information or even a second opinion if management questions arise. Where choices exist, do not be afraid to let your preference be known. On the other hand, if circumstances change, be willing to accept your obstetrician's advice, remain flexible, and change the "gameplan" if necessary. Remember, your doctor's concern is for your safety and that of the your baby.

Finally, take the pregnancy stories of relatives, friends and coworkers with a grain of salt. You are *you*, and you'll soon have your own tale to tell.

Suzanne G. Pratt, M.D., F.A.C.O.G.
The Three Rivers Gynecology, P.C.
909 North Fifth Avenue
Rome, Georgia

Introduction

Why is *This* Pregnancy Book Different from All Others?

"Why do we need another pregnancy book on the market?" This was my immediate response when I was asked to write this book. Well, after surveying the books that are already available, I came to a sorry conclusion: There wasn't the *right* information, all in one source, for the mid-1990s pregnant woman. In order to find out all you need to know about your health during pregnancy, you'd have to buy about 10 books! This didn't seem very reasonable to me, so I went to work and did a "competitive analysis" of all the pregnancy "products" I was up against.

After reading about 30 of the top pregnancy and childbirth books, I noticed some common information gaps. Most books devoted several pages or complete chapters to nutrition and recipes. Well, that's fine, but since all pregnant women should see a nutritionist to tailor their pregnancy diets to their individual needs anyway, shouldn't the space be used instead for less attainable information? For example, in some books, I found that more space was devoted to recipes than to abnormal bleeding!

I also noticed that many of the books devoted several pages to pregnancy symptoms in either a month-by-month or a week-by-week breakdown. Well, that's fine, too—or so I thought until I began interviewing a number of North American pregnant women. "I didn't suffer from *any* of the symptoms at the time I was supposed to" was a common complaint. "Nothing was mentioned about X or Y in the XXth week!" was another common complaint. Or, my favorite: "By the time I *found* the information I needed about a particular symptom, it was *gone!*" In other words, an easy-to-access, better organized list of symptoms was missing from the majority of pregnancy books out there.

And there was virtually no information at all on the subjects of high-risk pregnancies, common health problems during pregnancy, and the entire gamut of pregnancy loss issues, such as miscarriage (1 in 6 pregnancies ends in one) and ectopic pregnancy (there's an ectopic epidemic right now, thanks to the widespread incidence of chlamydia and gonorrhea). Instead, women who lost a pregnancy in the first or second trimester had to suddenly rush out and buy a "Pregnancy Loss" book. That seemed a bit rude to me. If I had a dollar for every woman who begged me to devote adequate space to miscarriage and abnormal bleeding in a pregnancy book, I'd be pretty rich.

Since most pregnant women work for a living and do brave battle in daily traffic jams, surely, I thought, someone had to have included *detailed* emergency childbirth instructions in a pregnancy book! I was wrong again. One page at the most was devoted to this in a few books, while most mentioned no emergency procedures at all. This is odd, considering how frequently 911 calls are made regarding emergency premature deliveries.

And what about a chapter devoted to finding good prenatal care to begin with for *this* decade? Or an entire chapter devoted to prenatal care for the high-risk pregnancy? Sex during pregnancy? Information about multiple pregnancies? Postpartum issues? *Correct* information about breastfeeding? Again, most of this information was either missing from the books or covered in superficial detail. Well, instead of babbling on about what I found sorely missing from the other books on the shelves, let me tell you about what's inside *this* one!

Chapter 1, "Your Pregnancy Management Team," contains everything you need to know about finding a childbirth practitioner (primary care physician, obstetrician, or midwife) and a birthing facility for your needs. What you need to be screened for when you're prenatal-care shopping, the questions you need to ask of your practitioner, and your rights and responsibilities as a pregnant patient are also covered here.

Chapter 2, "Everything You Need to Know About the 'High-Risk' Pregnancy" is exactly that. You'll find out if you're at "high-risk" during pregnancy, and, if so, the special care you need, the appropriate practitioners and the tests you can expect. In addition, the pregnancies that *develop* into high-risk pregnancies later on, as a result of gestational diabetes, toxemia, gestational hypertension, or thyroid disease, are also discussed in detail.

Chapter 3, "T1 Health (Trimester 1)," is all about your body in the first trimester. Included is an alphabetical list of every conceivable pregnancy symptom at this stage, as well as complete sections on yeast and urinary tract infections and a thorough section devoted to all the problems during pregnancy (miscarriage, ectopic pregnancy, bleeding), and detailed emergency procedures for dealing with these situations. And, of course, there is information on nutrition and fitness, too. (Oh, and in case the alphabetized symptoms lists fail in any area, I've got a backup plan: exhaustive cross-referencing throughout the book, as well as a detailed Index.)

Chapter 4, "T2 Health (Trimester 2)," is similar to chapter 3, but discusses mid-trimester symptoms and problems, including venous changes, water retention, and carpal tunnel syndrome. A large section on sex during mid-pregnancy is included, as well as information on prenatal exams and a discussion of things that can wrong at this stage, such as second trimester miscarriages, molar pregnancies, and a unique pregnancy-loss phenomenon known as "vanishing twin" syndrome.

Chapter 5, "Prenatal Testing," discusses ultrasound, alphafetoprotein testing, amniocentesis, and other prenatal tests. You'll learn about these tests, their benefits as well as risks, and about when they are necessary.

Chapter 6, "T3 Health (Trimester 3)," is similar to chapters 3 and 4 but also includes information on the baby's presentation or "lie," guidelines for childbirth preparation classes, and the range of problems that can occur at this stage, such as premature labor, false labor, and postmaturity. Antepartum fetal testing is also discussed here.

Chapter 7, "All About Labor and Delivery," is just that and talks about pain management, epidurals, fetal distress, episiotomies, surgical deliveries, cesarean sections, and more. It also includes a detailed section on emergency childbirth procedures, entitled "Childbirth 911". This section is designed to be copied and carried in your wallet so you can hand the instructions over to a taxi driver, coworker, salesperson, or whomever when you're caught off guard.

Chapter 8, "Health After Childbirth," covers hygiene instruction, postpartum symptoms, postpartum sex (Boy, does it ever change!), and contraception, as well as potential problems after childbirth, such as hemorrhaging and bacterial pelvic infections.

Chapter 9, "Breasts, Feeding and Other Milk Beefs," is entirely devoted to breastfeeding. It separates misinformation from the correct information and talks about common breastfeeding problems, breast infections, and breast self-examination (BSE).

Finally, chapter 10, "Postpartum Depression," demystifies this generalized label and explains the difference between postpartum depression, the maternal blues, postpartum psychosis, and a common physical condition called postpartum thyroiditis, which occurs in 10% of all postpartum women and is often misdiagnosed as postpartum depression. Symptoms and treatment for each condition are discussed in detail.

Now, there *are* some major issues that this book does *not* cover: fetal development and neonatal care (with the exception of breastfeeding) and specific information for the father. Why? I wanted to write a book for you and *you alone*. This book is about *your* body, during and after pregnancy. Fetal development and neonatal care are only discussed from the perspective of how they affect your body.

Prepregnancy planning, infertility, and fertility awareness are other issues not addressed in this book in detail. This book makes one *huge* assumption: you're already pregnant.

Discussion of abortion is limited only to information about the termination of a pregnancy in the event of a problem. I've made another huge assumption about you: Whether your pregnancy is planned or not, this is a *wanted* pregnancy.

So by now, you should have a pretty good idea of what's inside this book. And if the bookstore clerk isn't giving you the evil eye yet, I suggest you flip to the back for a list of alternative books you can read and organizations you can go to for more information. The idea is to give all the information you need about your pregnancy in *one source*. This is *your* pregnancy sourcebook: Use it, read it, and share the information with others.

1

Your Pregnancy Management Team

What do I mean when I say I want to address a *mid-1990s* pregnancy? We are in the midst of a second baby boom, but *this* baby boom is very different from the last one. The mothers are older, wiser, highly educated, and mostly professionals. As a result, the obstetrics "industry" has undergone radical changes. These consumers are more informed about health and nutrition than their predecessors; they are more concerned about maternal and fetal health; and they are questioning procedures and medications, and challenging the old pregnancy myths. But many are also under far more personal and financial *stress,* and are bearing children at a much older age than their "forebears." All this has led to a completely different picture for North American women giving birth in the mid-1990s and beyond. In addition, a new mythology has emerged as a result of the first crop of pregnant "boomers," which needs to be exposed. But before I can address the concerns of *today's* pregnancies, it's important to grasp the changes that have taken place. So, here's a brief 30-year history of pregnancy.

By the early 1960s, pregnancy research was rooted in comfort at the expense of the child; how to make the *mother* more comfortable—

with drugs—during her pregnancy and labor was the main intent. This kind of research yielded drugs that proved disastrous, such as thalidomide, a morning sickness (see chapter 3) drug that caused horrendous limb deformities in the children of the women who took it. DES (discussed in chapter 3), a more widely distributed family of drugs (taken to prevent miscarriage), was another such "comfort" product. And, of course, the entire labor-delivery process was sanitized. Surgical deliveries and cesarean sections were performed frequently; fathers were not involved in the birthing and delivery process at all; delivery rooms were sterile; drugs to "knock the mother out" during labor were standard procedure; forceps were commonplace; labor positions were tailored to optimize the *doctor's* comfort; breastfeeding was actually inhibited, as synthetic hormones were automatically given to the mother to halt her production of breastmilk (see below and chapter 9); postpartum depression was never discussed (see chapter 10); and mothers were taken by surprise by the hormonal changes and emotions they experienced after birth.

By the 1970s, the pregnancy mind-set had shifted about 180 degrees. Women were inherently more distrustful and suspicious of the entire pregnancy setup. Natural childbirth and home births flourished; breastfeeding was popularized; and men were initiated into the childbirth process as coaches and full partners. Meanwhile, another pregnancy issue surfaced that to this day is a passionate and difficult one: abortion. In response to decades of "powerlessness" in the delivery room, the women's rights movement, and a completely changing socioeconomic infrastructure, the mother's civil rights became the most significant pregnancy question of the 1970s. Legalizing abortion was more about regaining control over the pregnant body than it was about health; in short, it was (and still is) a *political* issue. (Mid-trimester abortion is discussed in chapter 5.) One of the products that emerged from this maternal civil rights war was the home pregnancy test kit. Women wanted the right to know *and* the right to privacy.

By the 1980s, more "right to choose" issues emerged: the right to choose children *and* a career, and the right to choose to have children after 35 was challenged—often simultaneously. Suddenly, women were demanding "prenatal value" from the health industry. They wanted to feel secure that their age and stress from their jobs were not damaging the fetus. They became more educated about nutrition during pregnancy to maximize their chances of bearing healthier children. Also, the era of prenatal testing emerged in the 1980s (a result of advances in technology), which is being further refined today. Another outgrowth of this decade was the growing importance of fitness during and after pregnancy. Because so many women were professionals, and more concerned with their postpartum figure than women 20 years prior, fitness became a significant issue in maternal and fetal health. (Unfortunately, both nutritional and fitness issues have developed into more of an obsession than a healthy concern, which I address in chapter 3.)

Finally, the concern with prenatal value was extended into the arena of labor and delivery. Home birth decreased in popularity because of all the normal complications that can arise during a routine birth. Women began to realize that, while home birth sounds very comforting, many women who gave birth prior to the invention of maternity wards died in childbirth. Hospitals have therefore become homier, and are no longer the sterile environments they once were. Today, technologies, delivery techniques, obstetric practices and behaviors, as well as medications, have been tailored to optimize both the mother's *and* child's health. And, of course, there is more postpartum value. Information about postpartum health and products such as breast pumps are more widely available, while political issues, such as maternity benefits, family leave, and quality childcare, have all extended into the legislation of the 1990s.

All of this has led to great changes and a different focus for today's pregnant woman. Currently, women account for about half of all practicing primary care physicians and obstetricians, which has helped "feminize" obstetrical care. Attitudes regarding the role of the traditional midwife have changed significantly; midwifery is now a certified, professional degree program at many universities across the Western world.

But there are unique issues in the 1990s that are affecting pregnant women dramatically. They revolve around a depressed economy; an STD-infected population; a sexually active preteen and teen population that has led to an increase in teen pregnancies (despite an increase in contraceptive education); a cancer-ravaged society; a weight-obsessed society, which contributes to eating disorders; a breast-obsessed society that has raised safety questions regarding "silicone breastfeeding"; an increase in the number of older women who are pregnant for the first time; an infertility epidemic (due in part to this increase); an environmentally toxic planet; and an increase in the incidents of multiple births, as a result of the widespread use of fertility drugs. This boils down to one word for pregnant women today: *STRESS*.

And since today the average planned first pregnancy occurs in women who range in age from 30 to their mid-40s, a considerably older pregnant woman is now the pregnancy novice. A first pregnancy in a woman under 30 seems the exception rather than the rule. This creates some concerns for the under-30 crowd, who may not need the same level of care as their older counterparts.

Since, as you may have heard several hundred times, no two pregnancies are alike, you'll need to understand how to *tailor* your prenatal care to your own needs, *prepare* for possible complications, and *plan ahead* for the most comfortable and appropriate labor and delivery conditions you can. And since, in the case of planned pregnancies, many first-time pregnant women have a more colorful gynecological and/or medical history than the generation before them, it's important to keep your medical history in mind when you're pregnant.

As many of us know, you don't need to actually go to see a doctor to confirm that you're pregnant; you just need to pop over to a pharmacy and spend about $20 on a home pregnancy test kit. At any rate, when the pregnancy is confirmed, women automatically assume that they need to immediately find an obstetrician, a doctor who specializes in prenatal care and delivery. Depending on where you live, this may not be necessary. First, not all women need an obstetrician. If you're under 35, are healthy, and have never had any significant health problems, you can, in theory, continue to see your primary care physician throughout your pregnancy and arrange to have him or her deliver your baby. The problem is, most primary care physicians in the United States don't practice obstetrics. In Canada, however, it's common for primary care physicians to handle all aspects of a routine pregnancy because they are trained in obstetrics. To date, obstetricians in the U.S. doubt whether the obstetrics industry will change even with the passing of health care reform legislation. If your primary care physician doesn't "do" obstetrics, you can see your primary care doctor throughout the first trimester, after which time you can be referred to either another primary care doctor who does obstetrics or an obstetrician for the remainder of the pregnancy. Your primary care doctor can also refer you to a midwife, which is a refreshing option for many women. A midwife can manage all of your prenatal care, delivery, and postpartum care. In this case, both the primary care physician and/or obstetrician can take a backseat, and only step in when there's a major problem. Often, all three practitioners work in partnership; the midwife "manages" the pregnancy, and the primary care physician and/or obstetrician are called in as "consultants" periodically just to make sure all is well. The role of the midwife as an obstetrics practitioner is discussed later in further detail.

The purpose of this chapter is to outline all the options available for excellent obstetrical care, the necessary screenings you should have had done prior to the pregnancy or as soon as you discover it, as well as define the pregnant patient's rights and responsibilities. Consider this chapter a crucial framework for making the most of your pregnancy and obstetrical management team from the outset.

The Pregnant Patient: In Search of Excellence

The only person more vulnerable than a woman in the Pap position is a pregnant woman in the Pap position (on your back in stirrups). That's why the most crucial aspect in planning your prenatal care is choosing a practitioner you're comfortable with over one who intimidates you.

Making the choice boils down to not only asking the right questions, but understanding how the pregnancy industry works.

A common misconception is the belief that *any* gynecologist will handle your pregnancy. It's not true. This obstetrical confusion is responsible for some very dissatisfied pregnant consumers. While all gynecologists are initially *trained* as obstetricians (hence the term OB-Gyn, which stands for obstetrician-gynecologist), not all gynecologists *practice* obstetrics. The reasons have to do with a combination of factors that include a maturing practice where the doctor's patients are finished with their families, and the doctor chooses a less frantic pace, as well the real dilemma of obstetrics liability. Because even the most routine pregnancy is "risky business," the cost of malpractice insurance significantly increases for doctors who practice obstetrics. These costs are more pronounced in the United States than countries with universal health care, but the insurance issue exists regardless of where you live. What about primary care physicians? Again, some primary care physicians do obstetrics while others don't; the reasons also often revolve around the insurance issue.

But regardless of whether your primary care physician practices obstetrics or not, finding good obstetrical care starts with finding good primary care first, and then a gynecologist who practices obstetrics. For any woman considering having children, obstetrics care should be a chief concern to raise when she's primary care shopping anyway.

The most important doctor-patient relationships a woman in her childbearing years can have are with her primary care doctor and obstetrician/gynecologist. Since most primary care physicians are qualified to practice basic gynecological care (pelvic exams and Pap smears) and routine obstetrical care, one would think that obstetrics and gynecological care is evenly split between OB-Gyns and primary care physicians. It isn't. In fact, 70% of the women who regularly see a gynecologist have *no* other doctor. More gynecologists are acting as primary care (i.e., overall care) physicians for women than family practitioners, for example, which can lead to problems. The confusion lies in determining what constitutes primary care for both the pregnant and non-pregnant woman. Primary care includes the following:

- an annual physical (routine screening for various diseases, such as diabetes, heart disease, or thyroid disease; checking your heart rate, blood pressure, and hormonal levels; conducting a urinalysis; and so on)—*most OB-Gyns will do only some of this;*
- an annual pelvic exam and Pap smear—*all OB-Gyns will do this (If your primary care doctor doesn't do pelvic exams on most of his/her female patients, this is a sign that he/she isn't as qualified to manage your basic gynecological care as a primary care physician who does. When the service is offered, however, this can be an ideal option.);*
- screening for and treating STDs (sexually transmitted diseases such as chlamydia, gonorrhea, herpes, etc.—see pages 21-23) and/or vaginal infections (yeast, trichomoniasis, etc.)—*all OB-Gyns will do this;*
- an annual breast exam (feeling your breasts for abnormalities)—*all OB-Gyns will do this;*
- monitoring your menstrual periods (keeping track of your periods and asking about irregular flows, missed periods, and so on)—*all OB-Gyns will do this;*
- counseling and medication (where appropriate) regarding nutrition, diet, family planning, health risks, and any other concerns you might have; OB-Gyns may just counsel you on family planning and direct gynecological/obstetrical health risks;
- checking out suspicious lumps, bumps, pains, irregular bleeding, or other suspicious symptoms—*OB-Gyns will do this only if the symptoms are gynecological-related;*
- referrals to specialists when necessary—*both OB-Gyns and primary care physicians will do this;*
- providing care for assorted aches and pains, colds, flus, viral infections, bacterial infections, and so on—*this is not an OB-Gyn's job, but when your infections are gynecological, he or she will treat them;* and . . .
- managing all aspects of a routine, low-risk, unremarkable pregnancy—*only gynecologists who practice obstetrics will do this; most internists in the U.S. will not;*

- providing basic pediatric care to your children, and calling in a specialist when necessary—*no OB-Gyn will do this.*

Meanwhile, general practitioners, family practitioners, and some internists will provide all of the services above. If they do not practice obstetrics, they will provide you with obstetrical care up until the fourth month of your pregnancy, then refer you to someone else.

Who is a Primary Care Physician?

If the road to an excellent obstetrician and/or midwife is through an excellent primary care physician, who is a qualified primary care physician? Seven out of 10 women will say a gynecologist is.

Gynecologists are doctors who specialize in caring for a woman's reproductive organs (her vagina, uterus, cervix, fallopian tubes, and ovaries) as well as her breasts (although most do not treat breast cancer). But are these the only parts that require care? Certainly, many gynecologists serve as excellent primary care physicians. A 1985 study found that, with the exception of cholesterol screening, OB-Gyns (obstetrician-gynecologists) performed what are considered primary care services for women on a more routine basis than traditional primary care physicians. During a routine visit, OB-Gyns were much more likely to do breast, pelvic, and rectal exams, cervical cancer screening (Pap smears), blood pressure checks, and urine testing than general practitioners (an M.D. with four years of medical school and one year of internship), family practitioners (an M.D. with four years of medical school and up to three years residency training in general/family medicine), or internists (an M.D. with four years of medical school and up to three years residency training in non-surgical treatment of several different illnesses). However, in a competitive industry, many gynecologists, as specialists, have been forced into a generalist role because of real financial pressure to keep women's primary care dollars in their pockets.

When you consider the fact that a gynecologist has only one year of training in general medicine and three years of training in obstetrics and gynecology, is it really wise to use a gynecologist for primary care?

A family practitioner and internist spends three or more years training to be a primary care doctor.

Women are caught in an ongoing debate between gynecologists and family practitioners. Many gynecologists argue that since they specialize in women's health, why does a woman need to go elsewhere? They are far more qualified to perform prenatal and gynecological exams than family practitioners (who may only have minimal training in these areas). The truth is that they specialize in women's *reproductive* health. What if you have a heart condition, diabetes, high blood pressure, epilepsy, or thyroid disease? Is the gynecologist more qualified to juggle all of these conditions when he/she is not trained for it?

Family practitioners, internists, and general practitioners, on the other hand, feel they are more qualified to assess the bigger picture, to juggle a cross-section of different health concerns, and to refer patients to a variety of specialists when necessary (including an obstetrician/gynecologist), and are certainly qualified to provide basic gynecological and obstetrical care—as they do for all other health areas. The fact of the matter is, a family/general practitioner's or internist's job is to act as your "general contractor," overseeing and project-managing your entire health scenario. Their specialty is to generalize and assess when to call in the *experts.* When it's time for a special job, they'll refer you to an obstetrician, gynecologist, nutritionist, endocrinologist, oncologist (cancer specialist), physical therapist, or whoever is needed. The bottom line is that an obstetrician-gynecologist is best utilized as a specialist, because that's what they've been trained as. So what's the solution? Become an educated health care consumer. Know what your doctor is qualified to handle before you register as a patient with him or her. That's why it's crucial to interview your doctor, using the questions outlined on pages 14–15. Here are two sample scenarios:

Plan A: Use Your Family Physician as a Basic OB-Gyn

Using your family doctor for *basic* gynecological and obstetrical care is just fine if you're healthy and have never had any gynecological or obstetrical complications before. (Past gynecological complications include endometriosis, pelvic cancer, positive Pap smears, STDs, and so on.) Past obstetrical complications include miscarriages, ectopic pregnancies, premature labors and/or deliveries, therapeutic abortions, and so on. In this case, your family physician will perform routine Pap smears and pelvic exams, provide you with contraceptive options, and advise you on family planning. When you're pregnant, if your history is unremarkable, your family physician can handle all of your prenatal exams, pregnancy discomforts, prenatal testing (if warranted), and labor and delivery. All of this is considered *primary care* for a sexually active woman.

Basic gynecological care is usually provided when you go for your annual checkup. You can also see your family doctor for "garden-variety" vaginal or vulvar irritations, yeast infections, and bladder infections (which are common in pregnancy). It is during an annual checkup that your family doctor will also check your overall health by conducting routine screenings (for cholesterol, hemoglobin, and hormone levels, etc.); taking a urine sample; checking your cardiovascular health, reflexes, eyesight, and hearing; and so on. As with any serious problem, your family doctor will refer you to a gynecologist or a gynecologist with a subspecialty if he or she finds anything abnormal in your gynecological exam, or feels you need a more detailed examination. These problems would include a positive Pap test, a particularly nasty yeast infection, an unexplained vulvar irritation, pelvic pain, difficult periods or irregular menstrual cycles, problems with fertility, irregular bleeding, and so on. If you're pregnant and are experiencing an unusual problem, your family doctor will also refer you to an obstetrician. The beauty of a family doctor is that he or she is trained to pinpoint the specialist you would need.

In many cases, a family doctor will immediately refer you to an obstetrician when you're pregnant, even if your pregnancy is routine and uncomplicated. This is simply because they lack the insurance necessary to practice obstetrics, as previously discussed. In fact, many American family doctors don't even attempt to practice obstetrics, even though they're qualified, to avoid the insurance risk, as do many American gynecologists. Yet in Canada and other countries with universal health care, family physicians will very often manage all aspects of a normal pregnancy and refer patients to obstetricians *only* when there's a problem.

If you have a more "colorful" gynecological medical history, so long as you've been treated successfully for your problem under the supervision of a gynecologist and have had three to six consecutive normal Pap tests and pelvic exams, you can resume basic gynecological and obstetrical care under your family physician. Your gynecologist should send your family doctor a *complete* record of your previous diagnoses, treatment, and current gynecological status. Then, your family doctor will be instantly alerted to any other problems. (In this situation, he or she may suggest that you remain in the care of your gynecologist for your basic gynecological needs anyway.)

There are several benefits of Plan A. First, your overall health will be better managed. Because family doctors are trained longer in general medicine (with the exception of a general practitioner), you'll receive better primary care with a good family doctor. Second, you'll have better access. You'll also develop a more intimate relationship with your family doctor. Family doctors are often more aware of your family medical history because they treat other family members, too. So they may be on the alert for certain symptoms or diseases that can affect your gynecological/obstetrical care. Finally, you may get a more balanced approach to healthcare. Family doctors see the big picture and tend to be less myopic about your healthcare.

Plan B: Separating Your OB-Gyn from Primary Care

This involves paying separate but equal attention to both your family doctor and OB-Gyn. Tell your family doctor that you have (or want to be referred to) an OB-Gyn who manages all your gynecological and obstetrical care and vice versa, but request that both doctors communicate about your health and report their findings on a regular basis. Then, if there's a health risk your obstetrician-gynecologist isn't taking into consideration when he or she recommends a certain treatment, your family doctor can be an extra backup. The benefits of Plan B are that you create a healthcare partnership between your family doctor and OB-

Gyn instead of a competition. Since each doctor is doing what he or she was trained to do, they work together to give you the best care possible, rather than competing. At the same time, you set up a system of checks and balances. If you have a question about your care, you can ask the other's opinion to confirm or alleviate your concerns.

Finding a Primary Care Physician

If you don't have a primary care physician yet, an American health insurance plan will have a list of primary care physicians you can interview. For uninsured Americans and any Canadian, you can find one the same way you find a good hair stylist: Ask your friends, neighbors, or relatives. Or, if you already have another specialist whose opinion you respect, such as a gynecologist, endocrinologist, oncologist, surgeon, chiropractor, or dentist, ask for the name of a good family doctor, who can then refer you to an OB-Gyn, when you need one (like right now, perhaps!). If this specialist is a woman, who is *her* family doctor? If this specialist is a male, who is his *wife's?* Once you find leads to a few primary care physicians, there are some basic guidelines you can use to select the one that's right for you.

1. *Do you like the way the business is set up?* Medical practices are organized in three basic types: solo practices (just the doctor and a support staff), partnerships (two or more doctors sharing patients, costs, and space), or combination/group practices (a collection of different specialists under one roof, who all work in a kind of team environment). There's no right or wrong setup, but the right choice for you has to do with what you're most comfortable with.

2. *What does your doctor call you?* Your doctor should call you by the name you're most comfortable with—be it a surname, first name, or nickname. It's more relaxing for both of you.

3. *Can you ask your doctor questions?* How open is he or she? If you can't question your doctor, that's a bad sign.

4. *Where is your doctor located?* Is the location convenient, or does

it take you over an hour to get there? Waiting to see the doctor is stressful enough, but if you're driving across the country just to go to your doctor, consider the stress involved with your appointments.

5. *Can you reach your doctor by phone?* Can you just pick up the phone and call him or her anytime to talk about a particular health situation? If you can't, is it because the doctor is truly busy or just not accessible after hours to patients? Doctors should leave an emergency number you can call after hours.

6. *If he or she weren't your doctor, would you want him or her as a friend?* If you wouldn't be caught dead having a cup of coffee with your doctor, why would you allow him or her access to your vagina?

When Do I Need an OB-Gyn?

You'll need an OB-Gyn if you're experiencing a high-risk pregnancy, as discussed in chapter 2. Generally, this means that you have a history of difficult pregnancies or pregnancy loss, you're carrying more than one baby, you're over 35, under 17, or you have some other health problem (gynecological or otherwise) that requires you to be expertly monitored during your pregnancy. The best way to find a good OB-Gyn is to be referred to one through your primary care physician. If you don't have a primary care physician, find one and *then* get referred to an OB-Gyn. For a more direct line to an OB-Gyn, you can also try the "hair stylist" route (see page 12) (although in Canada many OB-Gyns will not see you without a doctor's referral). Failing that, ask another specialist you're seeing for the name of a good OB-Gyn. Find out who that specialist's own OB-Gyn is, or, if he's a man, his wife's.

Are you new in town and don't know anyone? Call the American College of Obstetricians and Gynecologists (ACOG) at (202) 638-5577, tell them where you live, and ask them to recommend some names. In Canada, call the Royal College of Physicians and Surgeons. Do you have a particular condition, such as endometriosis, or fear complications during your pregnancy? Contact the self-help or nonprofit association/organization connected to your condition and ask *them* for names. Are you an immigrant? Perhaps you don't speak English very well? Contact your local ethnic association and ask if they have a list of doctors who speak Spanish, Korean, Cantonese, Japanese, French, and so on.

Finally, when you do find an OB-Gyn you like, whether on your own or through a referral, here are some questions you should ask the doctor when you go for your first visit:

1. *Are you board-certified?* This means that he or she has completed a residency training program that has met with the standards set by the American Board of Obstetrics and Gynecology. Note: OB-Gyns in their first 2–3 years of practice are Board-eligible, meaning that they simply haven't been out long enough to write the Board exams. If, however, they've been practicing over three years, and still refer to themselves as only Board-eligible, you should find out why they haven't yet written the exam!

2. *Are you board-certified in any subspecialty?* Does your gynecologist actually *do* obstetrics? You better check, because not all gynecologists do! Does he or she practice maternal-fetal medicine? And so on.

3. *What kind of hospital privileges do you have?* Full operating privileges are best.

4. *Do you share copies of medical records and test results with your patients at their request?* If he or she won't, that's a bad sign.

5. *Are you available for occasional phone calls?* Find out if the doctor is accessible, or if you have to make an appointment just ask him or her a question.

6. *What are your emergency arrangements?* If you suddenly find you're bleeding, does the doctor have a 24-hour emergency number, or a backup specialist if he or she is away?

7. *Is a female assistant present in the room when you perform a pelvic or prenatal exam? If not, do you object if I bring along a friend or my spouse?* If the male doctor performs solo pelvics, that's a bad sign, in some places, illegal.

8. *What's your philosophy on cesarean sections and episiotomies? What's your philosophy on hysterectomies?*
9. *How do feel about hormone replacement therapy? Abortion? At what age do you recommend annual mammograms?* All of these questions are important issues. The response you get will tell you about the doctor's ethics and flexibility, as well as expose his or her level of skill, education, and awareness regarding women's health issues.
10. *What kind of practice do you operate? Solo, partnership, combination practice?* Again, there are a variety of business setups your OB-Gyn may operate under, and you need to feel comfortable with it.

The Midwife

The pregnant patient has one more practitioner in the system she can turn to: the midwife. Even if you are experiencing a high-risk pregnancy, a midwife can manage all aspects of it. The best way to find a midwife is through either your primary care doctor or OB-Gyn. Either one will have a list of midwives they either work with or know through their professional networks. Although a midwife cannot offer you primary healthcare, in the U.S. she can perform routine pelvic exams and Pap smears, and manage basic gynecological care under the supervision of a gynecologist. She cannot substitute as a gynecologist when you're not pregnant, however; she is *solely* a pregnancy and childbirth practitioner.

Until this century, childbirth was considered "women's work" and didn't really involve men at all. Since biblical times, children came into the world with a midwife in attendance. Midwives had no medical credentials per se and were often older, "wise-women" in the community, or just real childbearing veterans themselves. Or they were aunts, mothers, sisters, good friends, and so on. When childbirth became "doctor's business" beginning around the eighteenth century, midwives were actually trained and became an integral part of the obstetrical industry all over the world, including Europe. (In fact the term *midwifery* was re-placed by *obstetrics* just this century.) Midwives have continued to rule the childbearing world across the globe, with the exception of countries practicing Westernized medicine.

In North America, until about the 1900s, all births took place at home with a midwife assisting. A doctor (a general practitioner) was on hand only if there was a problem or if a cesarean section was necessary. This might sound idyllic, but many women died in childbirth who never would have if given today's high-tech facilities and equipment, and many stillbirths were delivered that would not have occurred today. Many labors were also difficult, lasting as long as several days (which would never be allowed anymore). Midwives were also on hand for mis-carriages and other difficulties that occurred throughout a pregnancy.

Midwifery was never a recognized profession, however, the way nursing was. Even so, until the late 1940s, home births and midwives continued to dominate the childbearing industry, because many women were unfamiliar with the hospital birth. They were raised with certain assumptions about childbearing that stuck for a long time. In addition, transportation was difficult for many women who didn't have access to cars or who lived in more rural communities.

After World War II, as the baby boom and suburban living ex-ploded in the 1950s, the midwifery tradition pretty much died out. This left a significant hole in the childbearing process; midwives offered very important advice and emotional support throughout the pregnancy, which is now recognized as critical during labor, delivery, and the post-partum process.

In the 1970s, women's groups began lobbying to bring back mid-wifery and fought to have it recognized as a certified profession. The American College of Obstetricians and Gynecologists (ACOG) recog-nized midwifery as a profession in 1971, but it wasn't until the mid to late 1980s that midwifery finally became a certified professional graduate pro-gram at some universities in the United States. It hasn't taken long for women to welcome them back into today's childbearing process. In fact, midwives are thriving healthcare professionals very much in demand now.

How do I choose a midwife?

In North America, there are two types of midwives: a *certified nurse-midwife (CNM)* and an *independent midwife,* sometimes referred to as a *certified midwife (CM).* A CNM has a professional graduate degree in midwifery and has gone through more officially *recognized* medical training. A CNM always works *in partnership* with your managing practitioner. This means that she might manage your entire pregnancy and only refer you to a doctor if there's a problem. Or she may work right alongside your doctor and be with you for all your prenatal exams and tests. Many hospitals have CNMs on staff. If you're American, you may have a choice of CNMs on your health plan, just as you would a doctor. This care is covered by your insurance. Canadian women can choose CNMs through their hospitals or can contact the Ontario Association of Midwives at (416) 538-4389 to find out more about Ontario and Canada-wide services. This care is covered by the Province.

An independent midwife, or CM, has less official medical training, but usually has combined university courses with a type of internship or apprenticeship. These midwives are less likely to be covered by American health plans and would be paid for independently. For a low-risk, routine pregnancy, this midwife *is* qualified to act as the managing practitioner. She will also be able to refer you along the way to specialists, if you need them.

Hospitals and primary care physicians will have lists of both kinds of midwives. If you are a first-timer or are in a high-risk group, the best scenario is going with the CNM/physician team. Ultimately, whoever you choose will need to be interviewed (using the primary care physician guidelines on pages 12-13) and will need to have a personality compatible with yours. In some states, a *lay midwife* is also available, but she has absolutely no medical or academic training. She has apprenticed with another lay midwife who also had no medical or academic training. You may need to rethink this type of midwife.

It's also important to know how midwives add "value." Their role is to be a real friend to you throughout your pregnancy and to be a constant. They will help you through the discomforts of pregnancy and will be more available to you when you go into labor (which many doctors are not). They will also assist you in more emotional circumstances, such as after a miscarriage or when you hear bad news or learn about complications. They will be active in the postpartum period, and throughout your pregnancy will come to see you at home if you require immediate care. It's important to remember, though, that a midwife isn't qualified to manage complications during pregnancy, labor, or delivery; you'll need to be referred to an obstetrician under these circumstances.

Are you a midwife candidate?

Of course, midwives aren't for everyone. For one thing, depending on your health plan, you may not be able to afford one. Costs vary from state to state or province to province (midwives aren't fully covered by Canadian health insurance yet). Other reasons why a midwife might not be for you has to do with individual feelings; some women just aren't comfortable with the level of training a midwife has and feel more secure with the traditional specialist. Finally, you may feel comfortable with a midwife and would love to have one, but may already have the right standard of prenatal care in place through your primary care physician and/or obstetrician. In this case, a midwife may truly be an "extra" you just don't need.

The best thing to do if you're thinking about a midwife is to select a few to interview. Ask what services they can offer that your primary care physician and/or obstetrician can't. For example, midwives are trained in various massage techniques, natural remedies to help you cope with pregnancy discomforts, and so on. Find out how much a midwife costs. If, for example, the costs are lower than an obstetrician's, you might want to double up a midwife and primary care doctor. In either case, each practitioner is obligated by law to call in an obstetrician in case of a serious problem—that means you could still have the services of an obstetrician if you need one, but will benefit from a cost break if you don't.

Another important guideline for choosing a midwife has to do with how strong your support network at home is. Do you have supportive family and friends who can offer you advice and friendship during your pregnancy? How supportive (or available) is your partner? A midwife can offer crucial emotional support to you—something that many doctors can't. For more information, call The American College of Nurse-Midwives at (202) 728-9860. Canadians can call the number listed on page 17.

The Fundamentals of Obstetrical Care

Deciding on your prenatal management team is only half the task of the pregnant patient. You also need to coordinate a delivery team. You'll want to know who will deliver you if your own doctor is unavailable. The situation varies between your country's or community's hospital setup. For example, in Canada, if your own doctor is not available, you may wind up having whoever is on call at your birthing facility deliver you, a situation not as common in the U.S. That's why finding a good hospital or birthing facility is just as—if not more—important than finding good prenatal care. Finally, you need to understand when during your pregnancy you need to make all of these decisions, which leads us to the most confusing question of all: When should you first see the doctor?

For Planned Pregnancies . . .

Many women like to see their doctor after a positive home pregnancy test. They often request an "official" blood or urine test to confirm the results. With the high-quality kits on the market today, this really isn't necessary, but if it makes you feel better, do it. To figure out your due date, just count nine months plus one week from the first day of your last period (the beginning of your bleeding). For example, let's say the date of your last period was November 22. November plus nine months = August. 22 plus one calendar week = 29. Therefore, your due date will be August 29. Another way of calculating the due date is to simply *subtract* three months back and *then* add seven days: November minus three months = August, and 22 plus one calendar week is still 29—August 29.

When you go for your first prenatal exam (which is discussed in chapter 4), your doctor will just do the same thing, calculate a little room for error, and give you a rough date. That date is never a precise date. In fact, only about 5% of women actually give birth on their due date. A normal pregnancy ranges anywhere from 254 to 294 days! A typical scenario is preparing to deliver anywhere from two weeks prior to or past the due date. The *real* answer to "When should I see the doctor?" depends on the prep work you've done *before* the pregnancy. It also depends on your current health situation. Before you became pregnant, you ideally should have been screened for a number of conditions, diseases, and infections. The list is long, but includes all of the following conditions. For the purposes of completeness, information on treating many of these conditions is also included.

Several genetic disorders

There are numerous genetic disorders that you can be a carrier of, but not personally affected by. Some examples are Tay-Sachs disease (if you're Jewish or French Canadian), sickle cell anemia (if you're of Mediterranean or African descent); and certain diseases linked to the X chromosome (in other words, certain diseases carried by the female and passed on to her male child, such as various forms of muscular dystrophy including the leukodystrophies, hemophilia, and so on). When you present yourself to your doctor and tell him or her that you'd like to be screened for any possible genetic or chromosomal disorders, he or she will take it from there. Your race and family history will determine which diseases you need to be screened for. If you happen to be a carrier of a disease linked to the X chromosome, you'll need to go for genetic counseling, and weigh the risks, as well as prepare for various prenatal tests during the pregnancy (discussed in chapter 5). If you carry any genetic diseases that require *both* you and partner to be carriers before the genes can be passed on (such as Tay-Sachs disease, for example), then your partner must be screened as well. If you're both carriers, you'll also need genetic counseling.

Rh incompatibility

Your blood type is either Rh positive (meaning that you have an Rh factor in your blood, as 85% of us do) or Rh negative (meaning that you don't have an Rh factor). Either is fine, *but,* if your partner is Rh positive and you're Rh negative, your baby's blood type may not match yours. This can be a problem during delivery or even during a miscarriage or a therapeutic abortion. If you are a candidate for Rh incompatibility, your pregnancy needs to be monitored closely by an obstetrician.

German measles (rubella)

In early pregnancy, rubella can damage the fetus. 1 in 7 women have been vaccinated long ago for rubella, but may not remember it. You can be screened for a rubella titer, a test that detects whether antibodies to rubella are present in your bloodstream. If you have the antibodies, you're immune; if you don't, you'll need to consult with your doctor about steps to take next.

HIV (human immunodeficiency virus)

If you have reason to suspect that you've been exposed to HIV, you must take an HIV antibody test if you're either planning pregnancy or are already pregnant. (HIV and pregnancy is discussed in chapter 2.)

Chlamydia

Chlamydia is one of the STDs you'll need to make sure is treated before you become pregnant, or as soon as you discover you're pregnant. Ten percent of the time, people who have chlamydia will test negative for it. Chlamydia is one of the most common STDs in North America right now—in the sexually active 18 to 30 crowd, 50% have chlamydia. Chlamydia is particularly nasty because it is usually *asymptomatic* (meaning no symptoms). In one year, of the four and half million women in North America who will be infected with chlamydia, 60% of them will not have any symptoms. But the disease can do a lot of damage, leading to pelvic inflammatory disease (PID), as discussed in chapter 8. Some experts estimate that chlamydia causes 50% of all pelvic infections and 25% of all tubal pregnancies, due to scarring of the fallopian tubes. It can also cause urethral infections, cervicitis (inflammation of the cervix), and PID, which can lead to subsequent infertility or complications during pregnancy or childbirth.

The screening is simple. Your doctor takes a culture swab of cervical mucus. It can be done in conjunction with a Pap test. Chlamydia is *extremely* easy to treat: Tetracycline will cure it. The drug usually prescribed is called *doxycycline* (Vibramycin), which is a derivative of *tetracycline* (Tetracyn and many other brands). Two doxycycline capsules per day for 10 days will do the trick. Cheaper tetracycline must be taken four times a day, but many people forget to take that many pills; that's why doxycycline is better. If you're already pregnant, or cannot be on tetracycline, you'll be given *erythromycin* (Eryc, PCE, and many others).

As many as 10% of all pregnant women are believed to be infected with chlamydia. This can lead to all kinds of complications during pregnancy or at birth, including miscarriage or infant pneumonia, conjunctivitis (severe eye infection), or even blindness.

Gonorrhea

Gonorrhea is another STD that's pretty common and does more damage to women than men. However, it is *less* common than chlamydia. So, if you're diagnosed with gonorrhea, you'll also be treated for chlamydia. The reasoning: If she managed to catch gonorrhea, she's got an enormous chance of already having chlamydia. Better treat her for both just in case! In fact, a woman can often be simultaneously infected with both chlamydia and gonorrhea if her partner is a carrier for both infections. Women are thought to have a 30% chance of contracting gonorrhea after one sexual contact with an infected partner, and almost a 100% chance if they are on hormonal contraception. Like chlamydia, early stage gonorrhea is asymptomatic about 80% of the time. The occurrence of symptoms depends on where the gonococcal bacteria is *living*.

If you're having annual pelvic exams, your doctor will check your cervix for any unusual discharge and often take a culture for a routine screening. However, depending on what kind of test is performed, it may be unreliable. Usually, gonorrhea tests are 90% accurate if a culture test is done; if only a "gram stain" is performed, where the discharge is smeared onto a slide and stained, the test is only 50% accurate for women, but very accurate for *men with symptoms*. The best thing to do if you suspect you have gonorrhea is to request two culture tests one week apart.

If you *do* have gonorrhea, you will either be screened for chlamydia as well, or just treated for it anyway. In non-pregnant women, gonorrhea is easily treated with antibiotics as well: one dose of *ceftriaxone* (Rocephin one shot!) and a follow-up prescription of doxycycline to cure the probable chlamydia. If you're already pregnant, you'll likely be treated with ceftriaxone, but may be given another antibiotic safer for pregnancy. You'll need to discuss the risks of taking any antibiotics with your doctor and pharmacist. All hospitals now treat the eyes of newborns with silver nitrate or antibiotic drops to prevent gonococcal infection, just in case. Again, newborns can develop conjunctivitis if they're born to gonorrhea-infected mothers.

Herpes

Herpes is an STD caused by the herpes simplex virus. The virus enters the body through the skin and mucous membranes of the mouth and genitals, and then permanently sets up shop in the nervous system.

There are two types of herpes: herpes simplex virus type I (HSV I), which is characterized by cold sores and fever blisters on the mouth and face, and herpes simplex virus type II (HSV II), the dreaded genital herpes. Both I and II can erupt on the face or genitals, and either can be transmitted without intercourse. Herpes *is* contagious whether the sores are active or not. It is most contagious when the sores are active, but it's found that most infection takes place when the sores are *inactive*. This is when herpes is known to be asymptomatic. When the sores are active, they're visible and stand as a warning to the other partner *not to touch*. Indeed, touching the sores with your fingers and then touching the skin of a healthy person will transmit the virus. This means that it's possible for either facial or genital herpes to be transmitted on any infected person's fingers. That's how potent the sores are! When there are no visible sores, the warning isn't there, and the virus is also transmitted.

The herpes sores are called vesicles (pronounced vesickles), and they are painful, watery blisters that occur anywhere from two to 20 days after infection. Within a few days, the vesicles rupture, leaving behind shallow blisters that may ooze or bleed. After three or four days, scabs form and the vesicles fall off, healing by themselves without treatment.

There is no cure for herpes, but there are some antiviral medications (pills) that can help alleviate the pain of the vesicles. The initial outbreaks take longer to heal, lasting about two to three weeks. Then, the virus will start to taper off, and you may go from monthly initial outbreaks to just annual outbreaks. The usual pattern is nasty initial outbreaks, with milder episodes recurring within three to 12 months after the first herpes outbreak. Then, recurrences become milder and far more sporadic, like once every two years, and so on. Generally, factors such as stress, poor diet, caffeine, and hormonal elements (menstruation, use of oral contraceptives, etc.) trigger herpes outbreaks. The presence of other infections, such as vaginitis, genital warts, or yeast can also trigger a recurrence. Usually, there are fewer recurrences with HSV I. About 25% of people with HSV II may also never experience a recurrence.

Diagnosing herpes isn't difficult to do; when the sores are active, it's usually obvious. To obtain a definite diagnosis, a culture is recommended. A blood test can also detect whether you have herpes antibodies present. The problem with this test is that it can only tell you that there has been an infection at some point—not when it occurred.

Over 30 million North Americans are currently infected with herpes, but only about 25% of them know they have it. Its estimated that roughly 30% of the general population have been exposed to HSV II. If you've been exposed to herpes and are planning a pregnancy, ask your primary care physician for advice. The risk of passing on herpes to your spouse or partner years after an initial outbreak may be quite low if you don't suffer from recurrent herpes. Many women with herpes go on to have normal, healthy pregnancies and deliveries.

If you're already pregnant, make sure your obstetrical practitioners are aware that you have herpes. Depending on how frequent and severe your outbreaks are, you may need a cesarean section (discussed in chapter 7) to avoid transmitting herpes to your child—which is *very* dangerous. For the record, neonatal herpes is rare and occurs only in about one in several thousand deliveries. If you have recurrent outbreaks during your pregnancy, your baby has about a 3% chance of contracting it. Even in women who first contracted herpes during pregnancy, only about 40% of the babies born to those women will contract the virus.

For more information on herpes and pregnancy, contact The Herpes Resource Center (HRC), which operates a hotline: (919) 361-8488.

HPV: Human papillomavirus (genital warts)

Sometimes referred to as venereal warts, genital warts are also STDs. They are caused by the human papillomavirus (HPV). This virus is very similar to the one that causes skin warts, but there are over sixty types of HPV floating around. Warts are painless and can appear on the woman's vulva or cervix or on the man's penis. Unless the warts are on the cervix, your doctor can usually spot them and treat them with a solution that will burn the wart off. HPV on the cervix can take the form of raised or flat lesions. Both types of lesions will be picked up by a Pap smear; raised lesions are called *condyloma*. If left untreated, HPV can cause the cells on the lining of your cervix to change, which can lead to cervical cancer. HPV is currently *the* most common STD in North America. It is rampant in sexually active women aged 18 to 35. HPV can be treated but, technically, can never be cured. Once the warts are removed, the virus generally doesn't cause problems, but it remains in your bloodstream forever. Follow-up Pap smears for the first couple of years after an HPV diagnosis, and annual Pap smears after that, will enable you to nip HPV in the bud should it decide to erupt again. Treatment can encompass cryosurgery or laser surgery, or a sloughing cream that is applied to your cervix. Treatment during pregnancy will depend on how far along you are in your pregnancy, and how severe the genital warts are. Genital warts can be transmitted to the baby, however, and can even block vaginal delivery if they become extremely large.

Syphilis

Perhaps the most famous STD, syphilis was once a very serious, incurable disease of which "madness" was often the result. Today, it's easily treated with antibiotics. Syphilis is caused by a bacterium known as a *spirochete*. There are three stages of syphilis: primary, secondary, and tertiary (late stage). It's transmitted through sexual or skin contact with someone who is already infected. When you're pregnant, you can transmit the disease to your unborn child, which is dangerous and known as *congenital syphilis.* The number of congenital syphilis cases reported in 1988 was the highest since the early 1950s, and, in New York City alone, that number increased more than 500%! Untreated syphilis during pregnancy can lead to fetal bone and tooth deformities, fetal nerve damage, stillbirth, and fetal brain damage. All pregnant women should request a syphilis test, particularly if they're HIV positive. Syphilis spreads through open sores called *chancres* (pronounced shankers), or rashes that pass through broken skin or the mucous membranes lining the mouth, genitals, or anus.

In the 1970s, syphilis was virtually eliminated as an STD because it had been treated so aggressively in previous decades. However, in 1985, the incidence of syphilis began skyrocketing in the United States and has continued to rise.

Diagnosing syphilis is tricky. Known as the "great masquerader," syphilis symptoms imitate other disease symptoms and can be misdiagnosed. Syphilis is diagnosed through a blood test that checks for antibodies to spirochetes in the bloodstream. Two blood tests are involved: The first one screens for syphilis, and the second test confirms it. Syphilis is a miserable, damaging disease that is curable. It's treated with simple antibiotics, either penicillin or tetracycline. In pregnancy, tetracycline can't be used and is substituted with erythromycin. But—erythromycin isn't as effective as penicillin for treating the fetus. So, many pregnant women with syphilis will first be desensitized to penicillin, and then treated with penicillin instead of erythromycin. After you've been treated for syphilis at any stage, you'll need to have a follow-up test to make sure you've been cured.

Hepatitis B

Hepatitis B is a virus that causes inflammation of the liver. It's most common in women aged 15 to 39 and is a serious STD that is on the rise. It is transmitted through contaminated needles or blood (as is HIV), but it is also transmitted through saliva, semen, or vaginal fluid. *Mothers can also pass on this virus to newborns during childbirth.*

It can take up to 180 days after infection for any hepatitis B symptoms to develop. Most people who get hepatitis B remain well, have no symptoms, and completely recover. However, even if you're asymptomatic, the virus can cause damage to the liver, which can lead to serious illness and even death. Those who *do* get sick generally experience flu-like symptoms, jaundice, darker urine, and lighter stools. Generally, you will recover from hepatitis B, but if you're unlucky, the illness can overwhelm you for several months; you don't want to get hepatitis B if you can avoid it. Some people will always carry the hepatitis B virus and will remain infectious to others.

Unfortunately, there is no cure for hepatitis B, *but there is a vaccine!* In fact, safe sex is *not* considered adequate protection from hepatitis B; only a hepatitis B vaccine will protect you. Like HIV, hepatitis B can flourish in an anal sex "environment" and among drug users. However, tattooing, and ear piercing are also common routes of infection. Those at highest risk for hepatitis B are intravenous drug users, gay men, health-care workers, and prostitutes.

The hepatitis B vaccine is given by injection in three doses over a six-month period. The second shot is given one month after the first shot, and the third shot is given five months after the second. Other than a sore arm for a day or two, side effects from the vaccine are rare. If you do suffer from any side effects, you'll experience general feelings of "unwellness," such as fatigue. If this is the case, contact the physician or clinic that administered the vaccine.

Finally, if you have hepatitis B when you deliver, your baby can be treated for it by being bathed right at birth to remove all traces of your blood, and then vaccinated. In fact, it is now fairly standard practice for hospitals to vaccinate all newborns for hepatitis B, whether the mother was infected or not.

Mycoplasma

Mycoplasma (a.k.a. *Ureaplasma urealyticum*) is an asymptomatic bacterial infection that is more often than not, an STD. (In other words, virgins don't usually get mycoplasma!) Your doctor can detect mycoplasma by culturing cervical mucus during a routine Pap smear. It's important to be screened for mycoplasma prior to pregnancy because if left untreated, mycoplasma can travel to the endometrium, causing inflammation. This is known as *endometritis*—not to be confused with endometriosis. If you were pregnant with endometritis, the embryo may not implant in the uterus, and you would miscarry.

Vaginal infections

The most common vaginal infection is caused by the overgrowth of vaginal yeast known as candidiasis, which is discussed more thoroughly in chapter 3. Bacterial vaginosis and trichomoniasis are also common, and all three are characterized by an unusual, odorous vaginal discharge.

Trichomoniasis, known as "trich," is diagnosed by swabbing the vaginal discharge and examining it under the microscope. But trich can also cause urinary tract infections (UTIs), discussed next. Sixty percent of women with trich are cured with an antifungal medication called *clotrimazole* (Canestan). A higher cure rate is seen with *metronidizole*, given orally. In pregnancy, if you have no symptoms, treatment with metronidizole may be deferred until your second trimester as a precaution, but to date, no birth defects have ever been reported with this medication. Generally, if you're taking medication for trich, make sure your partner gets treated as well, because it can be passed back to you again and again.

For bacterial vaginosis, the treatment during pregnancy is clindamycin suppositories. If your partner has it, he should be treated with metronidazole. If he doesn't have it, make sure he wears a condom until you're cured.

Yeast and trich aren't dangerous to your baby per se, but could aggravate natural discomforts of pregnancy considerably. Bacterial vaginosis, however, can complicate your pregnancy if left untreated and can trigger premature labor.

Urinary Tract Infections (UTIs)

These are very common bacterial infections that afflict about 10% of all pregnant women. Inflammation of the bladder (cystitis) is a common UTI, and symptoms include painful and frequent urination. If left untreated, cystitis can lead to a more serious kidney infection known as *pyelonephritis*, which can cause problems for the baby. In some cases, pyelonephritis can develop without cystitis. It's more common for pyelonephritis to occur in the third trimester, when it can trigger premature labor. If you have a UTI, you'll be prescribed antibiotics that are safe to use during pregnancy. You should be screened, however, for the bacteria that causes cystitis *before* you become pregnant or as soon as you discover you are. This is done through a simple urinalysis.

Group B streptococcal disease

Group B streptococcus is a bacteria that normally lives in your vagina or rectum, along with a whole batch of other bacteria. Group B is a problem because it causes strep throat, scarlet fever, and some pneumonias. About 30% of all women are walking around with Group B "strep," but they don't necessarily have any kind of infection. Normally, this is just fine and doesn't pose any problems to your health, but when you're pregnant, it can cause serious problems either during pregnancy or after childbirth. If you have a history of STDs, have given birth to children infected with Group B, or have a history of premature labor, you're more likely to be a Group B carrier. To date, routine screening for Group B strep isn't done for numerous reasons that are too complicated to go into. What you should do is discuss your risk factor with your own doctor, and decide together whether you should be screened. Treatment will vary depending on your individual circumstances.

Autoimmune disorders

Autoimmune means "self-attacking." Many diseases that are hereditary, such as thyroid disease or diabetes, are autoimmune. When you're in your first trimester and early postpartum period, *your risk for developing an autoimmune disorder is at an all-time high!* This is because your immune system is naturally suppressed and *at an all-time low.* The body does this during pregnancy to protect the fetus, thereby avoiding a situation where your body "rejects" it, as it normally would with any foreign tissue. You should know your family medical history and the diseases that "run in the family," such as diabetes, rheumatoid arthritis, thyroid disease (Graves' disease or Hashimoto's disease), and so on, as well as the early warning signs of these illnesses. That way, if you have any symptoms your doctor can screen accordingly.

Full physical

You must have a full physical to make sure you have normal blood pressure, iron levels (to prevent anemia), blood sugar, urine (to prevent protein in the urine, as discussed in chapter 2), cholesterol levels, hormonal levels, heart rate, and so on. At this point, you should also discuss with your doctor whether you need booster shots for polio, tetanus, or diphtheria.

Did you do your homework?

If you've been screened for the above, you don't need to repeat these tests unless you have reason to believe you have contracted an STD, have a specific infection now, or have developed symptoms of an autoimmune disease.

If none of these tests were done, *don't panic!* All you need to do is see your doctor, tell him or her that you are X amount of weeks pregnant, and that you haven't been screened for anything yet. *Request a full physical and an STD screening.* He or she will take it from there. This will include everything discussed above. The screenings will be done via blood test, urinalysis (to check for urinary tract infections, sugar, or protein in the urine), Pap smear, and swabbings done during a pelvic exam. Most likely, the doctor will also do another pregnancy test since the blood is already taken. Then, call the doctor's office for your test results. If everything is negative (meaning "all clear"), you can discuss things like nutrition and diet with your doctor. He or she will probably put you on a vitamin supplement. And then, all you need to do is wait out the first trimester until you go for your first prenatal exam, which is discussed in chapter 4.

For Unplanned Pregnancies . . .

If your pregnancy was an accident, it's pretty safe to assume that you will *not* have had any appropriate screenings done. So this should be your first priority. You should also make sure you inform your doctor about the circumstances of your pregnancy and what type of contraception you've been using, if any.

Discovering the pregnancy will also affect each woman in dramatically different ways. If, for example, you're married and were using the withdrawal method combined with fertility awareness techniques, your pregnancy might be unexpected but not unwanted. If you're single and were actively preventing pregnancy, that's a whole different ball game.

If you have an IUD in place and still got pregnant or if you got pregnant while on oral contraception or other hormonal contraception, the situation needs to be addressed. If you had a casual encounter with a man and the condom broke, this will warrant an HIV-antibody test for sure. If you don't know who the father is, tell the doctor; if you weren't using any contraception, this needs to be addressed to avoid future accidents. You need to provide this information for your own protection and health. In many circumstances, free counseling, legal advice, and birth control and/or abortion counseling are available.

After all of these factors are considered, you'll then need to level with your doctor about your diet and lifestyle. Are you using drugs? Do you smoke? Do you drink alcohol? Do you normally practice safe sex? What is your medical history? What other medications are you taking? The condition of your ovaries, the progression of the pregnancy, and your answers to these questions will mean different things to the pregnancy, and in some cases, may warrant a *therapeutic* abortion.

What About My First Prenatal Exam?

You should have an initial prenatal exam as soon as you discover you're pregnant—anywhere between 6 and 10 weeks. Here, you'll be given a full physical and perhaps be screened for some of the conditions outlined above. Most important, the date of your last menstrual period—and hence, the pregnancy, can be more accurately established at this point. As we'll discuss throughout the book, dating the pregnancy accurately to begin with can avoid all types of problems later. At this first visit, you'll also be registered as a prenatal patient. Then, should problems develop, such as bleeding, and so on (see chapter 3), you'll have established a rapport with your doctor. From here on, you'll be seen about once a month. What to expect in a routine prenatal exam is discussed in chapter 4.

It's important to note that traditionally, the basic prenatal exam didn't take place until the end of the first trimester. Even today, many obstetricians (particularly in Canada) will not see you until you're at least 12 weeks pregnant. The high rate of pregnancy loss in the first trimester, coupled with the fact that the pregnancy was—until recently—viewed as too "early" for the doctor to really add any value to the patient, was what postponed the prenatal exam until this point.

But attitudes regarding when to have a prenatal exam are changing. Many doctors feel that the earlier you're examined, the better your pregnancy can be managed overall, preventing miscalculating your due date, poor nutrition, as well as missing the opportunity to screen for certain conditions. If your obstetrician is still using the "12 week" rule, you should be seen by your primary care physician when you discover the pregnancy. Then, at 12 weeks, you can graduate to your obstetrician if you need to.

Finding the Right Hospital

The most important decision you'll ever make as a pregnant patient concerns the *hospital* you choose for your delivery, *not the doctor.* For an unremarkable, routine pregnancy, the hospital will often make the difference between a good labor experience and a bad one. (Do bear in mind that if you live in a small town or less populated area, you may not have much choice when it comes to a birthing facility.) The biggest misconception many women have is the belief that their handpicked, Harvard-graduate obstetrician who looks after their prenatal care is the same doctor who delivers them. It doesn't work that way. Most doctors will *try* to be available for your delivery, but will warn you that they may not be and, ultimately, are often *not* available on the big day. The reason is simple: labor is unpredictable and most obstetricians' schedules are jam-packed. They are available for deliveries on a first-come, first-served basis. The exception to this rule is when you've prearranged a cesarean section or are being induced (for various reasons discussed throughout the book).

Primary care physicians are a little more likely to be available because they're not as booked up and are not exclusively seeing pregnant women. Midwives, however, usually are more available for delivery, which is perhaps the chief benefit to having one (as discussed on page 18).

If you don't have a midwife, and your doctor can't guarantee delivery, who *does* deliver you? In a teaching hospital, it will be whoever is on call in the OB-Gyn unit of the hospital when you go into labor. Actually, many women are rudely awakened to the fact that when all is said and done, chances are an OB-Gyn *resident* (a recently licensed general practitioner who is studying for a particular specialty, in this case, OB-Gyn) may wind up delivering them. In a community hospital, you'll be delivered by any physician or midwife on staff (not necessarily a resident). In some communities (particularly in Canada), if you go into sudden labor and need to be rushed to a hospital, whoever is on call in Emergency may deliver you if the hospital is short-staffed. In this case, you should be more concerned about finding a great hospital than finding a great doctor. But if you're seeing a private physician in a group practice, either your own doctor or another doctor in the group will attend to your labor. If you're seeing a doctor in solo practice, you may be delivered by one of the doctors who backs up him or her when he or she is unavailable.

Guidelines for choosing a birthing facility

You'll naturally want a hospital that has top-notch facilities, such as a neonatal intensive care unit and state-of-the-art fetal-monitoring equipment. But you should also *expect* to find a 1990s maternity facility that offers you choices, without a long, arduous search. For example, there are very few hospitals left in North America that *don't* offer the following:

- *Birthing rooms.* One-stop rooms where you labor, deliver, and bond with the newborn, after which you'll either be moved to another room to recover or may even recover in the birthing room itself.) This is preferable to a labor room followed by a separate delivery room. It's also much homier. These rooms are usually nicely decorated to mimic a home environment. Some U.S. hospitals now offer LDR (labor delivery recovery) or LDRP (labor delivery recovery postpartum) rooms. Today, U.S. hospitals are under pressure to discharge patients earlier and earlier. Women may give birth, recover, and return home in 24 hours or less. So you may either labor, deliver, and recover in one room, then transfer to a traditional hospital room for the remainder of your stay, or you may do everything in the same room until you check out.
- *Birthing beds.* These are adjustable, comfortable beds that allow you a variety of labor and delivery positions. The flat, 1950s gynecological exam-style beds with stirrups are not used anymore in a modern hospital.

- *Birthing chairs.* Ideal for the squatting-styled delivery. Squatting deliveries, discussed below, are *really* popular now.
- *Leboyer births.* Frederick Leboyer was a French obstetrician who advocated gentle, soothing deliveries that included warm baths for the newborns after delivery, immediate bonding with mom, soothing lights, and so on. Essentially, the days of whisking the baby away, immediately severing the umbilical cord, and spanking the baby to start his or her breathing are over! Most hospitals incorporate some aspects of this method; not too many go the whole nine yards, however.
- *"Rooming in" privileges.* Your baby stays in your room, and nurses are available around-the-clock to assist you in breastfeeding, bathing, and so forth. It's sort of like an "instant nanny" service at your disposal. You also have the option of *not* doing this.
- *Total father involvement.* No hospital will prevent the babys father from *complete participation* in labor and vaginal delivery. In fact, this is encouraged. Some hospitals may have a problem with his presence during a cesarean section. Just ask.
- *Total midwife involvement.* Some hospitals today offer midwife services, acknowledge midwifery as professional training, and welcome midwives into the birthing process. They're helpful, knowledgeable, and comforting.
- *Breastfeeding lessons.* There is currently a worldwide effort, led by UNICEF and WHO (World Health Organization), to make hospitals "baby friendly." This means doing away with and adopting practices that support breastfeeding in the hospital. In other words, a hospital in this decade should not only show you how to breastfeed properly but ensure rooming in, end the distribution of free or low-cost formula to new mothers in hospitals, not provide the baby with artificial nipples (which discourages breastfeeding), and so on. For more details, consult my book, *The Breastfeeding Sourcebook.*
- *Bathing baby lessons and baby changing lessons.* Someone will show you how to change diapers and bathe.

Note: Canadian women may need to shop around a bit more for certain facilities, simply because American hospitals are usually better equipped.

When choosing a birthing facility, some women may be concerned about certain archaic hospital practices they read about in various pregnancy books. Many of the things they warn you about aren't done anymore, including:

- *Shaving the pubic area before delivery.* Hospitals now realize that pubic hair is perfectly sanitary and doesn't need to be shaved. In fact, nicks and cuts in the area as a result of shaving are recognized as more hazardous.
- *Enemas before delivery.* You'll be given a choice regarding an enema if your doctor feels you need one for any reason.
- *Stirrups during labor.* Old-style stirrups are not used anymore, in the sense that you're involuntarily "tied down," but there are certainly foot supports available to help you bear down during labor. In cases where forceps are necessary (discussed in chapter 7), these foot supports are also helpful.
- *Synthetic hormone (bromocriptine in pill form) to suppress lactation.* This was used to inhibit the production of prolactin, necessary for the production of breastmilk. The benefits of breastfeeding have been recognized for a long time. The hospital will assume that you'll want to breastfeed unless you state otherwise. If you want to bottle-feed instead, or need to for medical reasons, speak to your doctor about it sometime before your due date. (Lactation suppression is still available for mothers who want it—see chapter 9 for more details.)

What you *might* want to know about the facility is the following:

1. Is the maternity unit well staffed at all hours?
2. What credentials does the on-call staff have in case you need to be delivered by one of them?
3. What is the hospital's philosophy regarding cesarean sections?

When are they done? Who does them? Are they open to vaginal births after a cesarean birth?

4. As a reference, can you contact a new mother who recently had her baby there?

5. What's the hospital's philosophy on *underwater birth?* This is a new process in which a baby is born in a kind of large jacuzzi-style bathtub. Some women really like this! Some hospitals have these facilities, others are concerned that the newborn might drown in the process—which is considered a very small risk by underwater-birth advocates. Although to date, underwater births don't add any proven benefits to the baby, it's helpful during labor and is soothing for mom.

6. What is the hospital's philosophy on *episiotomies* (a procedure in which the vagina is slit open a little to allow more room for the head to come out) or *epidurals* (a painkiller that numbs the pelvic region but doesn't interfere with labor). Both of these are discussed in chapter 7.

7. Does the hospital have board-certified lactation consultants on staff? This is crucial if you want to breastfeed. If the hospital doesn't, ask your midwife to recommend a consultant you can contact prior to the birth. See chapter 9 for more details. (Many midwives are also board-certified lactation consultants.)

Other Birthing Facility Options

You can also choose from a variety of maternity centers, which are generally staffed by CNMs and supervised by family doctors and/or obstetricians who remain on call for emergency situations or consultations. For routine, low-risk pregnancies, a maternity center may serve as an ideal option. Some maternity centers are even based within hospitals. The problem is, if you suddenly develop a complication at a freestanding maternity center, you may need to be transferred to a better-equipped hospital. To select a maternity center, use the same guidelines that are outlined above.

Finally, home birth is another option. After much thought, I've decided not to endorse this decision, simply because of the range of complications that can occur. However, in some states (but not in Canada), independent midwives (discussed on page 17) would be the practitioners appropriate for home care and home birth.

The Pregnant Patient's Bill of Rights

You're not just "eating for two," you're purchasing healthcare for two. Because of this, you have the right to participate in any and all decisions that involve you and your unborn child's health. The only time you waive this right is if there is a real medical emergency that prevents your participation. This means that, in addition to your usual rights as a pregnant patient, you now have the right to expect the following from your obstetrical health care provider:

1. Informed consent about any drug, procedure, or therapy, *prior* to administration. That means full disclosure about potential side effects, risks, or hazards to yourself or your unborn child.
2. Informed consent about all alternative therapies that could eliminate the need for drugs (such as epidurals) or obstetric intervention (such as episiotomies). You should be offered this information early in your pregnancy so you can plan ahead.
3. Full disclosure about the safety of *any* drug or chemical given during pregnancy, labor, birth, or lactation. In other words, no drug is considered absolutely safe during pregnancy and should, therefore, be avoided whenever possible. At the same time, there are many drugs that are considered safe during pregnancy whose benefit to you and your unborn child outweighs any risks. Treatment for STDs is an example of this.

4. Informed consent regarding the risks of all anesthetics in the event that a cesarean section is anticipated.

5. Full disclosure regarding a *new* drug, procedure, or therapy during pregnancy, labor, or lactation. In other words, if no documentation exists regarding its long-term or short-term potential risks, you need to know.

6. Full disclosure regarding the generic chemical name and brand name of any drug you consent to taking. That way, you can advise your doctor about any allergies you may have had in the past to such drugs.

7. Independent choice regarding medical decisions that affect your pregnancy. This means that should you consent to or refuse any drug, procedure, or therapy, you have the right to make your choice free of pressure or interference from any healthcare provider.

8. Full disclosure of the name and credentials of all your health-care providers. This means that anyone who attends you in a health-care setting must be willing to disclose his or her professional credentials to you, whether they're residents, nurses, medical students, or candy stripers. If you're not satisfied that they're sufficiently trained, you have the right to refuse treatment from them.

9. Full disclosure as to the purpose and level of urgency of any drug, procedure, or therapy. In other words, is the therapy being done for your benefit or the baby's? Is it an emergency, elective, or experimental therapy?

10. The right to companionship during your labor and delivery. You have the right to bring anyone into the delivery room with you as a labor partner, whether it's your spouse, sister, or next-door neighbor!

11. The right to choose the most comfortable and least stressful position for labor and birth. This means that the practitioner who is delivering you should bow to your preference regarding position, whether you're squatting, sitting, lying down, and so on, unless there is a medical reason.

12. The right to care for your baby at your bedside, as long as the baby is healthy, and the right to feed the baby according to your and your baby's needs.
13. Full, written disclosure of the name and credentials of the person who delivered the baby. This information should also be on the birth certificate.
14. Full disclosure of the health of your baby.
15. The right to have complete, unaltered, uncensored, and legible hospital and medical records for you and your baby retained by the hospital and offered to you or your adult child before they are destroyed. In addition, you have the right to access these records whenever you wish and to obtain a copy of them.

Whether you're pregnant or not, you have the right to expect the following from your health care providers:

- *As much information as you want.*
- *Time to address questions and concerns.* If your doctor doesn't have the time to answer your questions, you should be able to call him or her or make another appointment that serves as a question & answer period.
- *Reasonable access.* You and your doctor must decide together what "reasonable" means. Do you need scheduled weekly, monthly, quarterly, or annual appointments? Or do you just want to see the doctor when you feel like it? How far in advance do you need to book an appointment?
- *To participate in the decision-making process.* To do this, you'll have to ask questions and be willing to educate yourself about your condition.
- *Adequate emergency care.* Who looks after you after hours when your doctor is sick or on vacation? Is there a substitute doctor?
- *To know who has access to your health records.* How confidential are your health records? Can your doctor release them to just anyone—your employer, insurance companies, government

authorities, and so forth—without your permission? What are your doctor's legal obligations with respect to health records, and what are yours?

- *To know what it costs.* If you live in the United States, you have the right to know what your bill will be in advance. Get an estimate and have the doctor break down each charge so you know exactly what you're paying for and what your insurance plan will cover. If you live in Canada, make sure all appointments, tests, and procedures are covered by your Province before you consent to anything.

- *Be seen on time.* If you're on time for an appointment, your doctor should be as well. Do you generally have to wait more than 30 minutes in the reception area before your doctor will see you?

- *To change doctors.* Yes, you can fire your doctor. If you're unhappy with your current doctor, or simply need a change, you have every right to switch. Make sure you arrange for your records to be transferred!

- *A second opinion or a consult with a specialist.* If your doctor is unable to make an adequate diagnosis, you can insist on a referral to either another doctor or a specialist.

The Pregnant Patient's Obligations

Finally, not only are you purchasing healthcare for two, you're *responsible* for two! This means that you need to be proactive about your obstetrical care by:

1. Educating yourself. Learn about the physical, psychological, and emotional processes involved with pregnancy, labor, and postpartum recovery.

2. Learning about all your obstetrical care options and choosing the practitioners appropriate for you.

3. Informing yourself about the hospital policies and regulations that will affect your labor, delivery, and postpartum recovery. Arrange for a tour, and so on.

4. Arranging for a companion or support person to help you during your pregnancy, labor, and delivery.

5. Calmly and clearly making your preferences known at the beginning of your pregnancy to your obstetrical care team regarding maternity care, prenatal testing, alternative therapies, or objections to certain procedures.

6. Researching the costs of your care in advance (not as necessary for Canadians).

7. Notifying your practitioners of your intent to seek care elsewhere and *identifying* your reasons for changing.

In addition, whether you're pregnant or not, your healthcare provider is entitled to the following:

- *Full disclosure.* Practitioners aren't mind readers. If you're withholding information about your family's medical history, your prescription drug use, addictions, allergies, eating disorders, specific symptoms, and so forth, it's unfair to expect an accurate diagnosis. Also, your doctor could prescribe a drug that you're allergic to or one that conflicts with other medication.

- *Common courtesy.* Treat your healthcare providers like business associates. If you make an appointment, show up on time; if you need to cancel, give 24 hours' notice.

- *Advance planning.* Plan your visit in advance, and think carefully about your symptoms. Don't go to your practitioner with a vague complaint like you're "not feeling well" and expect a full diagnosis. When you make an appointment, tell the receptionist how much time you think you'll need for a full examination, and write down your symptoms before your visit. Give the doctor something to work with.

- *Questions and interruptions.* If you don't understand something, ask. Interrupt the doctor, if necessary, and ask for a simpler explanation of what's wrong. If you don't do this, you can't blame your doctor for not giving you enough information.
- *Follow advice and follow through.* Take medication as directed and follow your doctor's advice. If you're experiencing side effects to a medication, have a problem with his or her advice, or your condition has worsened, let the doctor know. Full disclosure is important.
- *No harassment.* If you need to talk to your doctor, go through reasonable channels. Use the after-hours emergency number the doctor leaves with the answering service, or call your doctor's office during business hours. Don't continuously call the doctor at home at 4:00 in the morning, and don't call the office 10 times a day with every little ache and pain.
- *Enough time to make a diagnosis.* Diagnoses don't happen overnight. Allow the doctor enough time to examine you, run necessary tests, and so on. This might mean that you need to wait longer for an appointment so your doctor can schedule enough time to fully examine you.
- *Room for disagreement.* What you think is in your best interest may not be what your doctor thinks is best. Allow for a difference of opinion and give your doctor a chance to explain his or her side. Don't just leave in a huff and threaten to sue. Maybe your doctor is right.
- *Professional conduct.* Don't request unusual favors that compromise your doctor's moral beliefs, and don't ask your doctor to do something illegal (i.e., writing bogus notes to your employer so you can claim disability pay).

Incidentally, if even a few of these responsibilities are abused, your healthcare provider has the right to resign and request that you seek care elsewhere.

Now that you've got your obstetrics team in place and know your rights and obligations as a pregnant patient, it's time to start your self-education. Read on to find out all about pregnancy: how it feels, what to expect, how to cope with a potential problem, and everything else I've included in the next nine chapters.

2

Everything You Need to Know About the "High-Risk" Pregnancy

A high-risk pregnancy sounds far more ominous than it really is. As you'll see below, you can be in excellent health and be labeled "high risk" from the moment you discover you're pregnant, solely because of your age or past obstetrical history. In other cases, women who have a chronic health condition such as diabetes or multiple sclerosis will also be considered high risk because there are more potential problems that could arise. You also can begin as a routine pregnancy and become high risk if you develop certain problems or conditions as the pregnancy progresses.

Unfortunately, when you're told that you have a high-risk pregnancy, you'll naturally be more anxious about the outcome. But you can also welcome the news as an advance warning, something to which not all pregnant women are privy. *In other words, women who have a high-risk pregnancy should perceive the extra care they'll be receiving as a bonus, not a burden!* If you're a high-risk pregnancy, you'll have more opportunities to catch and correct a potential problem than women who are considered routine pregnancies.

The purpose of this chapter is to calm you down, not raise more concerns You'll find out about the spectrum of high-risk pregnancies, all the doctors you'll need on your obstetrical team and how they will provide you with extra care, the tests you'll need to have throughout your pregnancy, and the purpose behind all this extra care.

Your Obstetrical Credit Rating

The best way to think of "high risk" vs. "low risk" labeling is as an obstetrical credit rating. When you seek financing, a financial institution will naturally look at your payment history, check to see if you've ever declared bankruptcy, check your current assets, and so on. They'll then classify you as either a high-risk or low-risk borrower. A woman who went bankrupt ten years ago, who is currently running a successful business and earning six figures, is considered a riskier borrower than a woman who has been working in the same middle-management position for 10 years, never missed a credit card payment, yet who is earning under $40,000 per year. Obviously, the first women is in better financial shape, but her bankruptcy sticks out like a red flag to any potential lender.

Obstetrics works the same way. Each obstetrics patient is evaluated for risk factors that predate the pregnancy.

The point is, the high-risk label does not necessarily mean you are in poorer health than a woman who is considered routine or low risk. It simply means that you are starting your pregnancy with a statistical red flag—more things tend to go wrong with women who have your red flag than women who don't. Red flags that aren't present in early pregnancy may develop later on, which I will discuss further in this chapter.

The Red Flags

Your pregnancy is considered high-risk if you:

- are over 35 years old (because of the risk of Down's Syndrome);
- are under 17 (more things can go wrong because you're not fully developed at this point);
- are having a multiple birth;
- have a history of chronic gynecological problems, such as pelvic inflammatory disease (PID), endometriosis, large, symptomatic fibroids, and pelvic cancers (a yeast infection, treated STD, or UTI does *not* make you high risk);
- have a history of breast cancer or cancer therapy;
- have a chronic health condition that requires ongoing care, such as diabetes, blood-clotting disorders, and heart problems;
- have a history of troubled pregnancies (repeated miscarriages, an ectopic pregnancy, premature births, stillbirth);
- have the potential of passing on a genetic disorder to your child, or have already had one child with a genetic disorder;
- have an STD;
- are pregnant as a result of assisted conception techniques;
- have ever had an abortion;
- are a DES daughter; or
- have an IUD still in place.

That's a pretty long list, but, as I'll go into further on, most of these conditions simply require a little extra monitoring. This type of high-risk pregnancy differs from a routine pregnancy that become high-risk when a woman develops a specific condition or infection *during* the pregnancy, which requires treatment and/or monitoring (discussed further below).

Who manages a high-risk pregnancy? That depends on your red flag. In general, the rules for a higher risk *early* pregnancy don't change, except in this case: you *will* definitely need an obstetrician, not just a primary care physician. You may also need a *perinatologist* (an obstetrician who subspecializes in high-risk pregnancies). You'll follow the same steps in terms of screenings and so on, as outlined in chapter 1, but as the pregnancy develops, you may need to take greater care than a low-risk pregnant woman. You will also need to undergo more prenatal testing. To better understand how each specific red flag affects your prenatal care, let's discuss them one by one.

Age

If the only reason you've been labeled high risk is because you're over 35, one difference between your prenatal care and a routine patient's is that you'll be recommended for *amniocentesis* (discussed in chapter 4). You're also more at risk for hypertension and diabetes. This is because there is a higher risk that your baby may have a chromosomal defect, the most common of which is Down's syndrome. You may also require more ultrasound tests than a routine patient. If the idea of amniocentesis bothers you, there is an alternative called chorionic villus sampling (CVS), a test that is performed in the first trimester. (See chapter 5 for more details.) The only doctor you absolutely require on your team is a good obstetrician. (See chapter 1.) You should also have an alpha fetoprotein (AFP) screening done, which checks for neural tube defects in the fetus.

If you're under 17, you'll also need an obstetrician. Depending on how the pregnancy is going, you may need to have certain prenatal tests performed.

Multiple-birth pregnancies

Multiple births seem to be back in vogue. In the 1950s, twins naturally occurred in 1 out of every 80 pregnancies. That number dropped by the 1970s to 1 out of every 100 pregnancies. Today, however, fertility drugs have caused the incidence of multiple births to skyrocket: *7 of every 100 pregnancies are twins; 5 of every 1,000 pregnancies are triplets; 3 of every 1,000 pregnancies are quadruplets; and quintuplets—once exceedingly rare—occur in 1 of every 1,000 pregnancies.*

Carrying more than one fetus presents some special challenges that you need to be aware of. Technically, you can determine whether you're carrying twins in the second month through blood tests and ultrasound. However, you may not know that you're carrying more than one fetus until the second trimester, because the pregnancy may seem quite routine.

Early detection is important because the gestation period for a multiple birth is shorter than with a singleton. A single-fetus pregnancy is about 40 weeks long, but with twins the pregnancy tends to last only 37 weeks, while triplets are born after about 35 weeks. The more fetuses you're carrying, the higher the chance of premature labor. Carrying more than one child also means that your risks of low birth weight, birth defects, and cord problems are especially high.

The risk of pregnancy loss also increases as does the risk of developing other pregnancy problems, such as *toxemia* (see page 65) and *autoimmune disorders*. If you have an existing red flag that marks you high risk from the outset, that condition can be exacerbated creating a "very high-risk" pregnancy. Finally, the delivery of the second twin is another unique consideration (see chapter 7).

As a result of some of the risks associated with carrying multiple fetuses, some couples in very high risk situations are opting for a procedure known as "selective reduction." Here, one or more fetuses is aborted to save the life of one or more fetuses in utero. This is a situation reserved for women who are in danger of losing all of their fetuses preterm. Usually, this situation arises after an assisted reproductive technology procedure where multiple embryos are transplanted into a woman's uterus. In some cases, this situation arises in women with a history of difficult pregnancies and pregnancy loss. If you feel you are a candidate for selective reduction, you'll need to discuss all of the risks involved with your obstetrician.

To manage a multiple-birth pregnancy, you'll need an obstetrician as well. In addition, you'll need to have a pediatrician who subspecializes in neonatal medicine chosen and "waiting by the door" for your first twin to be born. (Your obstetrician should refer you to a pediatrician sometime in the second trimester, since you're likely to deliver prematurely.) You will probably need several ultrasounds throughout the pregnancy but will not need a maternal serum alpha fetoprotein screening. You won't need amniocentesis unless another condition warrants it. If you do deliver prematurely, you may need to be transferred to a hospital that handles premature newborns, and a neonatologist may need to be consulted.

Because of the special needs of the multiple-birth pregnancy, I've provided separate sections on multiple-birth pregnancies in chapters 3, 4, 6, 7, 8, and 9. Check them out.

Other gynecological problems (PID, endometriosis, fibroids, history of pelvic cancers)

Past episodes of PID (pelvic inflammatory disease) are generally not a problem once you're pregnant. If you had episodes of inflamed fallopian tubes (salpingitis), for example, the fact that you're pregnant means that the inflammation wasn't severe enough to prevent conception. You may be more at risk for an ectopic pregnancy, which you should discuss with your doctor. PID could also cause inflammation of your cervix (cervicitis), which may lead to problems during delivery. Chapter 1 discusses STD screenings in detail. For more information on PID, see appendix A at the back of this book.

As for endometriosis, pregnancy—believe it or not—causes endometriosis to go into temporary remission, because you don't ovulate when you're pregnant. Furthermore, permanent remission of endometriosis has been known to happen after childbirth. The endometrial growths, in this case, shrink, and the pain associated with the disease stops. That being said, women with endometriosis have a higher risk of ectopic pregnancy and miscarriage. One study has found that the full-term pregnancies and labor of women with endometriosis are more difficult. If you have endometriosis, you'll need to be under the care of an obstetrician and be closely monitored for any bleeding or symptoms of ectopic pregnancy. Otherwise, unless you're over 35 or have another red flag condition that warrants prenatal tests, you'll just require ultrasound testing and monthly prenatal checkups beginning before month 4. Be sure to watch out for pains that appear unusual and bladder and/or bowel problems.

If you're pregnant with fibroids, you should be monitored by an obstetrician who has managed other fibroid pregnancies. *Intramural* fibroids (growing in the muscle layer) and *submucosal* fibroids (growing within the uterine cavity) are the most troublesome during pregnancy.

These kind of fibroids can change the shape of the uterus or interfere with the placenta's blood supply. If the fibroids were small prior to conception, the increased amounts of estrogen and progesterone coursing through your system during pregnancy can cause the small, never-before-bothersome fibroids to grow, which could trigger a late miscarriage or premature labor. Frequent checkups and monitoring will be necessary. Larger fibroids can sometimes obstruct the birth canal, meaning that you'll need to deliver by cesarean section. Other than an ultrasound and the routine prenatal tests, you shouldn't need any extra tests done unless you're over 35 or have another red flag condition.

If you have a history of cervical, vaginal, or vulvar cancer, cervical dysplasia, or genital warts on your cervix, so long as your condition was successfully treated, your pregnancy will not be any more vulnerable than a routine pregnancy. Other than seeing an obstetrician, your prenatal care will remain routine, unless you have an abnormal Pap smear.

History of breast cancer or cancer therapy

If you have had a history of breast cancer, let's assume that you've discussed the risks of pregnancy with your breast surgeon, medical oncologist, and radiation oncologist. Once that's done, so long as your breast cancer is in remission, your pregnancy should progress normally and you'll simply need to be under the care of your obstetrician. You'll also need to continue performing BSE (breast self-examination), even if your breast(s) was/were removed. You'll also need to discuss the risks of breastfeeding.

If you first discover breast cancer *while* you're pregnant, your pregnancy will progress normally, but your breast cancer may progress more aggressively since the extra blood flow to the breast and hormonal changes in your body can feed the cancer. Essentially, every case carries unique considerations regarding treatment and pregnancy. For example, your treatment may begin after you deliver, or for some women who are diagnosed in very early pregnancy, abortion may be a recommendation and treatment may begin immediately. It depends on the kind of cancer, the stage it's in, stage the pregnancy is in, and your own feelings regarding treatment. You can also breastfeed your child from a cancerous breast, so long as chemotherapy or radiation treatment hasn't yet begun. You'll need to discuss your treatment options with a breast surgeon, medical oncologist, radiation oncologist, and obstetrician trained in the disciplines outlined in the paragraph above.

For any other cancer histories prior to pregnancy, such as Hodgkin's disease and leukemia, you, too, should have discussed the risks of pregnancy with your medical oncologist and radiation oncologist (but often radiation oncologists do not require follow-up appointments after treatment). During the pregnancy, you may need to be monitored by your medical oncologist or radiation oncologist in addition to an obstetrician. This translates into monthly visits with your obstetrician and visits with your oncologist(s) once every trimester or so.

Chronic health conditions (diabetes, asthma, rheumatoid arthritis, multiple sclerosis, thyroid disease, and heart problems)

First, let's assume that you've already discussed pregnancy with the specialist who manages your condition. Then, in addition to either an obstetrician or a perinatologist trained in maternal-fetal medicine, you should be monitored by your regular specialist (i.e., an endocrinologist, cardiologist, or pulmonary specialist) just as often. You'll need to see each physician once or twice a month throughout the pregnancy. You may need to adjust your medication throughout the pregnancy, get extra rest, eat special foods, be treated if your condition worsens, and so on. *Finally, you must see a nutritionist during the pregnancy* (your OB-Gyn or perinatologist can refer you) *to tailor your diet to your specific condition.* Your prenatal tests, however, shouldn't differ from those of a routine pregnancy unless you have another red flag condition that warrants more testing or you develop complications related to your existing condition.

Some conditions actually improve during pregnancy. Seventy-five percent of pregnant women with rheumatoid arthritis experience an improvement in their arthritis symptoms during the first trimester. The symptoms become even milder as the pregnancy progresses. However,

90% of women with rheumatoid arthritis will experience more severe arthritis symptoms *after* delivery. Other research shows that if rheumatoid arthritis runs in your family, becoming pregnant at a younger age may reduce the risk of developing it in the first place.

When it comes to lupus, which is common in young women, if the disease is in remission at the time of conception, there's a risk that you'll experience a relapse. However, many of these relapses can be managed successfully, and your baby can be born without any complications. Nevertheless, you do need to follow the guidelines above, seeing your own specialist in addition to an obstetrician.

First developing a health problem during pregnancy, such as gestational diabetes, high blood pressure, toxemia, or thyroid disease, is a bit of a different ball game. This is discussed in the next section, which also outlines the questions to ask.

A troubled obstetrical history (repeated miscarriages, difficult pregnancies, an ectopic pregnancy, premature births, and stillbirths)

Let's assume that you've either corrected an underlying problem responsible for your past obstetrical history or know for a fact that your problem(s) resulted from unknown causes. Once that's clear, you can start anew—it's a new fetus and new pregnancy with new odds. You'll still need to see an obstetrician who is familiar with your history. You'll need to have regular ultrasounds and, depending on your history, other prenatal tests. A crucial point to make for women with a history of ectopic pregnancy: so long as the risk of another ectopic is ruled out at the beginning of your pregnancy, your risk factor for the duration of the pregnancy essentially evaporates. Once the fetus implants itself in your uterus, you're no longer considered a "high-risk" patient unless you have another red flag condition, or you develop a problem later on in your pregnancy.

If you have an *incompetent cervix*, which is discussed more in chapter 4, you'll need to have your cervix closed up until you're ready to deliver. Your obstetrician can do this anytime in the early second trimester and sometimes later.

At risk for passing on a genetic disorder or have already had one child with a genetic disorder

Let's assume that if you're at risk, you've gone for genetic counseling. If you haven't, do it now! You'll need to be managed by an obstetrician who possibly specializes in maternal-fetal medicine, but this greatly depends on the problem. Often, an additional specialist, who in this case would be a neonatologist, may not be called in until after the baby is born. You may also want an obstetrician who performs therapeutic abortions, should you want one, but often if you opt for an abortion, you'll be sent on to an abortion clinic. As for a genetic counselor, you'll probably be referred to one if haven't seen one yet. You'll also need to have a neonatal specialist chosen by the second trimester. You'll need to undergo ultrasounds, chorionic villus sampling and/or amniocentesis, and maternal serum alpha fetoprotein screening.

STDs

Review the section on STD screening in chapter 1. Also review the section on page 59 on red flag viruses.

If you're HIV positive

There are a number of factors that pregnant, HIV-positive women need to consider. First, progesterone during pregnancy induces a state of natural immunosuppression, which prevents the mother's body from rejecting the fetus, which is really a "foreign" object that presents potential danger to the immune system. Interestingly, during the last months of pregnancy, there is a decrease in the number of infection-fighting T4 cells in the body, which also occurs in HIV infection. Whether or not a further reduction in T4 cells to an already immunosuppressed woman speeds up the progression of HIV to AIDS is not known. It is suspected, however, because disease progression in HIV-positive women advances in pregnancy. This has yet to be proven.

Ironically, HIV infection does not seem to affect the course of pregnancy itself. But if you're pregnant with full-blown AIDS, you will be at risk for all kinds of viruses and other infections that can affect the pregnancy. Giving AZT to an HIV-positive woman in late pregnancy can dramatically decrease her baby's chance of being infected. No increased risk of birth defects has been reported in "AZT babies," except for a mild anemia at birth. However, the most profound impact of HIV infection on pregnancy is the *outcome*. Children born to HIV-positive women have a *30–50% chance of being infected with HIV.* If an HIV-positive woman delivers a baby who has not been infected, *the child can still be infected through breastmilk.*

If you are HIV positive and in your first trimester or fourth month, you should definitely consider having a therapeutic abortion. If your pregnancy has progressed beyond this, you'll need to see an obstetrician who specializes in maternal-fetal medicine as well as an infectious disease specialist. As for prenatal testing, so far, amniocentesis does not detect HIV infection in the fetus. There are three good reasons why amniocentesis isn't performed on HIV-positive women: First, the procedure can potentially expose the baby to the virus. Second, there is no real benefit of amniocentesis to the HIV-positive prenatal patient, and finally, there are some risks that the procedure poses to the healthcare provider.

Ultimately, whether you terminate a pregnancy or carry it full term, you should consider *permanent* forms of contraception to prevent a future tragedy like this. HIV-infected children can be subjected to extremely sorrowful lives, particularly when they're given up for adoption (which happens a lot) or are orphaned. It's found that many HIV-positive women progress to AIDS shortly after delivery. If the children are survived by their parent(s), the impact of their suffering and deaths deeply affects the family.

Infectious disease specialists recommend that HIV-positive women combine safe sex with permanent sterilization to avoid conception.

Assisted conception

If you're pregnant as a result of *clomiphene citrate* (Clomid) or other fertility drugs, you have a greater risk of having a multiple-birth pregnancy. Therefore, make sure you have an ultrasound in the early first trimester to rule out or confirm a multiple-birth pregnancy. (See the section on multiple pregnancies above.)

If you're pregnant as a result of artificial insemination, your pregnancy is no more risky than a routine pregnancy. If your pregnancy resulted from *in vitro fertilization* (IVF), *gamete intrafallopian transfer* (GIFT), or other technological procedures, you have a higher risk of miscarrying. You should definitely be seeing an obstetrician trained in reproductive endocrinology. Your tests will include regular ultrasounds and maternal serum alpha fetoprotein sampling; you shouldn't need amniocentesis unless another condition calls for it.

History of abortion

The risk of future complications from a legal abortion is small. However, there may be complications involving the cervix, and for that reason, your obstetrician must know about your abortion history. It's also worth noting that you can have your care managed by a primary doctor or midwife. You won't need any special tests or procedures unless you run into roadblocks later on.

You're a DES daughter

Any woman born in the United States from 1941–1971 (and perhaps even later) may be a DES daughter. During this period, five million pregnant women took the drug *DES (diethylstilbestrol,* a synthetic estrogen) to prevent miscarriage. Any daughter born to a mother who took DES runs a higher than normal risk for reproductive organ abnormalities, cervical and vaginal cell changes, and cancer. All this can spell trouble during pregnancy. If you are a DES daughter, you'll need to have all of your prepregnancy gynecological needs handled by a gynecologist, rather than a family doctor. In pregnancy, you'll need an obstetrician trained in gynecologic oncology to manage your pregnancy. You'll also need to have a special DES pelvic exam and Pap smear, where cells from all corners of your vaginal wall and cervix are annually investigated.

DES was administered under a host of different labels. If you can, find out the name of the drugs your mother took during her pregnancy and contact DES Action at 510-465-4011. Ask them to check if any of the drugs you discovered match the drugs on their list. DES Action has a nationwide referral service to doctors who specialize in the treatment of DES-exposed women.

If you're a DES daughter, you'll need to discuss with your doctor the risks that your particular physiology can pose to your pregnancy.

If you have an IUD still in place

This can put you at high risk for an ectopic pregnancy. Since the IUD cannot prevent an ectopic pregnancy in the way that an oral contraceptive can, if you're an IUD wearer who accidentally got pregnant, the chance of that pregnancy being ectopic is greater. If a fetus does implant itself in your uterus, you'll need to get your IUD removed ASAP. If the IUD is left in, your risk of a uterine infection is extremely high, and can even be fatal. You'll need to be under the care of an obstetrician in this case and watch for signs of ectopic pregnancy, as discussed in chapter 3.

Questions to Ask

All of these histories and/or chronic conditions mean different things in the case of pregnancy and carry special concerns and warning signs. Although your questions will vary with respect to your condition, here are some key questions to ask:

1. How will the pregnancy affect my current condition?
2. How will the treatments I've had in the past (lasersurgery, chemotherapy, radiation, other surgical procedures) affect my pregnancy and fetal development?
3. How will my condition affect labor and delivery? For example, if I had treatment for cervical dysplasia five years ago, can I still expect to have a vaginal delivery?
4. What kind of symptoms am I likely to experience because of my medical history?
5. What warning signs should I be alerted to during the pregnancy?

6. How can I contact you should something go wrong?
7. What can I do during the pregnancy to avoid any of these symptoms? (bed rest? diet? vitamin supplements?)
8. Any activities I should refrain from to maximize my health during pregnancy? (For example, sexual intercourse may be safe for some women and not for others.)
9. What sort of prenatal testing do you plan for me and why?

Again, whatever your medical history, you should also contact the specialist who usually *manages* your condition and see him or her regularly during your pregnancy.

From "Routine" to "High Risk"

Pregnant women can, of course, get sick with a cold or flu bug, just like any nonpregnant person. *Getting sick with a cold or flu does not mean that your pregnancy has suddenly become high risk.* You'll need to see your obstetrician or pregnancy practitioner at any rate, and follow his or her advice. *Warning: Do not take any medications unless your practitioner advises it.*

Certain viruses, such as *cytomegalovirus, toxoplasmosis,* and various STDs, *can* pose danger to the pregnancy or newborn. Depending on the severity of the virus and when it was caught during the pregnancy, you may or may not develop into a high risk. These viruses are discussed in the next section.

As mentioned in chapter 1, if you have a history of autoimmune disorders or a family history, you may need to be screened, but this depends on whether you're displaying symptoms.

Finally, there are other common health problems that develop in pregnancy that don't seem to be hereditary, but rather seem to strike "arbitrarily." Most of these conditions are manageable, but will change a routine pregnancy into a higher-risk pregnancy, in which case you'll need to be monitored by an obstetrician and possibly a specialist. For any number of problems, you may need to take certain medications, adjust your diet, or be on bed rest. Unfortunately, even in a book devoted to pregnancy, it's not possible to list *every* conceivable condition that can develop during pregnancy, so I'll discuss some of the more *common* problems that you might be concerned about. In addition, review chapter 1, which discusses the important conditions you'll need to be screened for before or in the early stages of your pregnancy. If you haven't been screened for the conditions listed in chapter 1, STOP READING AND DO IT NOW! Then come back and read on.

"Red Flag" Viruses

Life on planet Earth means that we are exposed to countless viruses and bacteria on a daily basis. Most of these viruses will not affect your pregnancy, but there are a few that you should be aware of.

Sexually transmitted diseases (STDs)

Just because you've been screened for these in early pregnancy doesn't mean you can't contract one after! *If you've had unprotected sex with more than one partner since your last STD screening, go back and get re-screened!* You can be given antibiotics safe for pregnancy to cure chlamydia, gonorrhea, and syphilis. As for herpes, review the herpes section in chapter 1; you may need to deliver by cesarean. Undiagnosed chlamydia and gonorrhea can cause a range of problems for you and your baby.

Treatment depends on how progressed the STDs are and how far along you are in your pregnancy. A final note: *Has your partner had unprotected sex without your knowledge since your last STD screening?* This might be a question to ask him if you're concerned.

The human papillomavirus (HPV), which causes genital warts, is another very common STD that may be picked up by a Pap smear. If you contract this during pregnancy, treatment may be able to wait until you deliver. There is also a danger that the warts can block the birth canal.

For chlamydia, gonorrhea, syphilis, herpes, and hepatitis B (which there is a vaccine for, as discussed in chapter 1), you'll need to be treated by an obstetrician and possibly by an infectious disease specialist, if you have a particularly nasty case. You may also need to undergo amniocentesis to see if your baby has been infected by your STD.

As for HIV, you can develop it in pregnancy if you have unprotected sex with an infected partner. If you have reason to suspect this is a possibility, get tested. Review the section on page **54** on HIV; you may need to consider a therapeutic abortion.

Toxoplasmosis

This ancient parasite is fast becoming a major concern for pregnant women. This is a protozoan that's contained in the feces of some cats, which can be dangerous to persons who are immunosuppressed: pregnant women and people who are HIV positive. Women in their first trimester are more vulnerable to toxoplasmosis, but if you're a cat owner, you may have already developed antibodies to this parasite, and hence, will be immune to toxoplasmosis. Nevertheless, if you have a cat, or have been around cats prior to conception, *ask to be screened for toxoplasmosis antibodies (via a simple blood test).* If you have antibodies, it means that you're immune to the infection; if you don't, it means you're vulnerable to the infection. In this case, if you have a cat, it's not necessary to board it in a kennel or with friends until you deliver, but by all means, avoid the cat's litter box and wash your hands after petting it! If you don't own a cat, avoid the homes of people who do until you deliver.

Cats can be tested for it, but it can take several weeks for it to show up in your cat. Outdoor cats are more likely to carry toxoplasmosis; they get it from eating mice. Poorly cooked pork or lamb may also carry toxoplasmosis. Common symptoms are swollen lymph nodes, fever, and fatigue. This virus is often mistaken for mononucleosis, but only 1 in 1,000 pregnant women will contract toxoplasmosis, while only 1 in 10,000 babies are born with congenital toxoplasmosis, of which only a few will develop serious problems. If you do find out that you've been infected, you'll need to see an obstetrician who may consult a maternal-fetal medicine specialist as well as a genetic counselor, but congenital toxoplasmosis isn't usually diagnosed until birth. There are tests that can be performed that can detect whether your baby has been infected.

Cytomegalovirus (CMV)

I had planned a long section on this virus because I noticed all the space other pregnancy books devote to it. After consulting with my medical advisors, and investigating all of the data and statistics about CMV, I've concluded that it's a shame so many women have been scared to death about this infection.

The bottom line about CMV is that about 80% of the general population is immune to it. Of those who aren't already immune, it's only dangerous to women who are pregnant or those with a lowered immune system (who should be more concerned about other viruses than CMV). The greatest risk CMV poses is to women who are infected with the virus for the first time. But even then, the virus is almost impossible to detect because the symptoms are vague and common cold-like. This creates the problem of realistically and practically screening women for CMV. To date, most doctors will not bother since those at true medical risk represent an exceedingly tiny segment of the population, coupled with the fact that there is no treatment for CMV. In short, the chances of CMV posing danger to you during pregnancy is about the same as contracting leprosy during your pregnancy. Almost nil. There are plenty of other things you can spend your time worrying about.

Chickenpox (varicella)

Like German measles (rubella), the chickenpox virus *can* cause birth defects during the first 16 weeks of pregnancy and complications for the newborn. If you've already had the chickenpox (and 85–95% of all adults have), don't worry about it; you're immune. If you've never had chickenpox, stay away from anyone who has either chickenpox or shingles, which is related to the varicella virus, because it can make you sick during pregnancy and, in extreme cases, even lead to pneumonia. If your newborn has been exposed, the baby will be treated with an injection of varicella-zoster immune globulin (VZIG). The herpes medication *acyclovir*

(Zovirax) may also be given intravenously to a newborn to increase protection if it's suspected that the fetus was exposed to chickenpox. In general, though, even when the fetus *is* exposed to chickenpox during the first trimester, *there's only a 2–10% chance that any birth defects will develop.*

Common Health Problems in Pregnancy

Family medical histories tend to rear their ugly heads when you're pregnant. For example, if diabetes runs in your family, you have an increased chance of developing *gestational diabetes* (diabetes during pregnancy). If thyroid disorders run in your family, you may develop a thyroid problem either during pregnancy or after delivery. The same rules apply to hypertension, which is often the first symptom of a more serious condition, known as *toxemia*.

Gestational diabetes

When your pancreas can't produce enough of the hormone *insulin* to metabolize sugar, you become diabetic. Sugar will build up in your blood, causing your body's entire metabolism to radically change. Pregnant women are particularly susceptible to diabetes, because during pregnancy, the placenta produces several hormones that counteract the effects of insulin. The body is therefore forced to produce as much as 30% more insulin than it normally does. Women with a family history of diabetes are more vulnerable, while women who have pre-existing diabetes may find it more difficult to control their blood sugar.

Diabetic pregnancies need to be expertly monitored because diabetes can lead to numerous problems during pregnancy and labor. But women who already *know* they're diabetic have been monitoring themselves all their lives; they administer their own insulin, carefully watch their diets, and are well acquainted with their condition. It's important for a diabetic patient to carefully plan her pregnancy when her diabetes is under tight control, which will decrease the risk of any related birth defects. In addition, meticulous management of diabetes during pregnancy appears to decrease the risk of stillbirth and/or complications related to having a large baby.

This is *not* the case for women who only first *develop* diabetes during pregnancy, known as *gestational diabetes*. This may be only a temporary condition, correcting itself after delivery, *or it may develop into a permanent form of diabetes after delivery*. Gestational diabetes tends to occur later in the pregnancy, and is discovered when a routine urinalysis (performed during a prenatal exam) reveals excessive amounts of sugar in the urine. You're more prone to gestational diabetes if you:

- have a family history of diabetes;
- previously gave birth to a baby over nine pounds;
- suffered from unexplained pregnancy loss;
- are over 25 years old;
- are overweight;
- have high blood pressure;
- are susceptible to repeated yeast infections (discussed in chapter 3).

Today, all pregnant women should be screened for diabetes, which entails two tests. The first test is called a *glucose screening test*. This involves reporting to the doctor's office at your convenience at some point in the second trimester. You'll be given a specified amount of sugar water, and then have your blood sugar tested an hour later. If it comes back abnormal, you'll go on to have the more formal glucose tolerance test. It should be noted that just because you have an abnormal glucose screening, doesn't mean that you automatically have gestational diabetes, which is why a more formal test for the condition is done in this case. A *glucose tolerance test* involves eating normally for three days, then fasting for at least eight hours overnight. The next morning, you'll report to the doctor's office and have your blood sugar levels measured to establish a baseline, after which you'll drink a specified amount of sugar water. Your blood sugar is then measured 30 minutes later, then hourly for about five hours. These readings will determine whether you *truly* have gestational diabetes or not. If you do, you'll be placed on a special diet and will need to have *frequent* urine and blood tests done throughout your pregnancy to monitor your blood sugar levels.

Just as there is more than one type of diabetes in nonpregnant people, there is also more than one type of gestational diabetes. Type I, or insulin-dependent diabetes mellitus (IDDM), is when insulin must be injected daily to control blood sugar levels. Occasionally, gestational diabetes will take the form of Type I and may become a permanent condition. Usually, gestational diabetes is Type II, or non-insulin-dependent diabetes mellitus (NIDDM), in which diet can control the blood sugar levels. Again, this type of gestational diabetes may either correct itself after delivery or may become a permanent condition. It's also important to note that Type II diabetes may *at times* require insulin injections to compensate for dietary laziness. Eighty-five percent of all diabetics have Type II.

The diet for insulin-dependent diabetic women includes between 2,200 and 2,400 daily calories, divided into 45% carbohydrates, 25% protein and 30% fat. The gestational diabetes diet (regardless of type) is similar. It will be monitored by either an obstetrician or even a perinatologist and/or an endocrinologist. Following this diet will be the key to a normal pregnancy; when blood sugar levels are normal in diabetic women, there are no more complications during pregnancy than in that of the general population.

If the condition remains uncontrolled, however, a condition called *ketoacidosis* can develop. This is when an increased acidity in your body creates an acidic fetal environment, which can cause impaired fetal growth or fetal death. If repeated urine and blood tests show abnormally high blood sugar levels *despite* a controlled diet, you'll be admitted into the hospital and be treated intravenously with insulin therapy.

Gestational hypertension (high blood pressure)

During early pregnancy, blood pressure levels normally decrease, but then they begin to steadily rise during the second and third trimesters. If your blood pressure was high prior to your pregnancy, you have what's known as *chronic hypertension;* if you only first develop hypertension after the first 20 weeks of pregnancy, you have *gestational hypertension.* You're more likely to develop gestational hypertension if you:

- are experiencing a first pregnancy;

- have a kidney disease;
- have diabetes (chronic or gestational); or
- practice poor nutrition.

Gestational hypertension usually clears up after delivery, so the treatment is usually lifestyle-adjusting therapies: bed rest, good nutrition, and frequent checkups. If your diastolic blood pressure (the bottom half of the fraction) is over 100, you may need antihypertensive medication to control the problem.

Women with chronic hypertension tend to have a family history of hypertension. They also tend to be:
- over 35;
- smokers;
- overweight; and/or
- suffering from a kidney disorder.

Whether you have chronic or gestational hypertension, high blood pressure in pregnancy could also be a symptom of *preeclampsia*, a serious condition discussed below, placental problems, or oxygen problems. Generally, most pregnant women with chronic hypertension will be managed with medications that control their condition. To be safe, if hypertension runs in your family, make sure you have your blood pressure levels checked *prior* to conception and frequently throughout the pregnancy.

Toxemia

Toxemia comes from the Greek words *toxikon,* meaning "poison," and *haima,* meaning "blood." This umbrella term is used to describe *four separate* and distinct conditions:
- *Preeclampsia.* This is a condition that comprises three symptoms that all trigger one another: water retention, high blood pressure, and protein in your urine (called *proteinuria),* which can lead to (or be symptomatic of) kidney damage. If you have only one or two of these symptoms, *you don't have preeclampsia!* All *three* of the above symptoms must be present in order to be diagnosed with preeclampsia.

- *Eclampsia.* This is a more severe form of preeclampsia in which in addition to the three symptoms listed above, you may suffer from epileptic-like seizures. Usually, preeclampsia is caught and treated early enough to prevent eclampsia. But if you *do* progress to this, hospitalization and possibly premature delivery by cesarean section may be necessary.
- *Gestational hypertension.* In the past, toxemia was used interchangeably with the term *gestational hypertension,* which is a separate condition (discussed just above) that, by itself, is *not* preeclampsia *or* eclampsia, but can be a symptom of either one.
- *Severe water retention.* Again, in the past, the term toxemia was used interchangeably with the term water retention. Water retention, by itself, is *not* preeclampsia *or* eclampsia, but can be a symptom of either one.

If you're told you have toxemia, find out *exactly* what your symptoms are. In almost all cases, a diagnosis of toxemia means preeclampsia. If you have seizures you have eclampsia.

Preeclampsia tends to occur in the later months of pregnancy, but it can be diagnosed as early as the fifth month. It's usually seen in first pregnancies and is more likely to occur in:

- women with hypertension (gestational or chronic);
- women with a kidney disorder;
- women with diabetes (chronic or gestational);
- women who are underweight or overweight;
- women carrying multiple fetuses;
- women under 18; and
- women over 35.

One of the most obvious signs of preeclampsia is a rapid weight gain, caused by an unusually high increase in bodily fluid. This is pretty easy to diagnose; you'll be suffering from extreme water retention (also called *edema),* which makes the joints around your hands and feet very puffy and swollen.

If your water retention isn't brought under control, the added fluid in your body causes your kidneys to secrete a hormone known as *renin,* which, in turn, increases your blood pressure. Once this happens, kidney damage may occur (which is diagnosed through protein secretions in the urine), after which you can retain even *more* water!

How is all this "water damage" treated? Some believe that a low-salt diet helps to bring water retention under control, but many doctors now think that salt intake has nothing to do with water retention at all. Bed rest is usually recommended. If your condition worsens, you may need to have certain prenatal tests performed to check on the fetus's health, be hospitalized, or, in a worst-case scenario, may need to be delivered prematurely possibly by cesarean section. A perinatologist may need to be called in to manage your condition, but usually an obstetrician can successfully treat preeclampsia and/or eclampsia.

Thyroid disease

Your thyroid gland is a butterfly-shaped gland located around your windpipe. Its job is to make thyroid hormone necessary for regulating every cell in your body by extracting iodine from various foods. About 1 in 20 persons worldwide suffers from thyroid problems, which occur about 5-7 times more frequently in women. Many thyroid problems are hereditary and are an *autoimmune* ("self-attacking") disorder. Again, when you're in the first trimester and the early postpartum stage, your risk of developing an autoimmune disorder is at a lifetime high; if thyroid problems run in your family, you're likely to encounter one during your pregnancy.

The most common thyroid diseases are Graves' disease and Hashimoto's disease. With Graves' disease, the thyroid gland becomes overactive, causing you to become *hyperthyroid,* or to secrete too much thyroid hormone. In this case, your body speeds up: Your heart rate might soar to something like 180 beats per minute; you might feel hot all the time; you may experience diarrhea, weight loss, and profuse sweating; you may develop what's called a *goiter,* a visibly enlarged thyroid gland that swells out of your neck. With Hashimoto's disease, the opposite occurs: you become *hypothyroid*, or secrete too little thyroid hormone. Here, your body slows down: the symptoms include a slow pulse, extreme fatigue, feeling cold, weight gain, puffiness, water retention, constipation, and dry skin—a little more like overall pregnancy symptoms. In this case, you may also develop a goiter.

Thyroid problems are diagnosed in pregnancy through a simple blood test and can be managed by both an obstetrician and an endocrinologist. If left untreated, they could lead to miscarriage, stillbirth, and fetal or congenital thyroid diseases. To treat Graves' disease during pregnancy, you'll be given *propylthiouracil*, a daily antithyroid medication that is safe for pregnancy. Graves' disease often improves as the pregnancy progresses, and your medication dosage will be lowered accordingly. To treat Hashimoto's disease, you'll be given a daily pill of thyroid replacement hormone, which replaces the hormone your thyroid has stopped producing. This medication will not harm the baby in any way and will cure your hypothyroidism. Sometimes Hashimoto's disease improves as well, in which case your thyroid medication dosage will be adjusted. Postpartum thyroid disease, sometimes misdiagnosed as postpartum depression, is discussed in chapter 10.

The best way to control thyroid disease during pregnancy is to know your family's medical history so you can be diagnosed early. Oddly, if you have premature gray hair, you're statistically more likely to come from a thyroid family. If you are a thyroid disease candidate, request regular thyroid function tests throughout the first trimester of your pregnancy and after delivery.

I hope all of this high-risk pregnancy material didn't scare you away, but for those of you who *are* high risk or may develop a high-risk pregnancy later on, it's important to know about *how* various conditions affect your pregnancy, and what to expect in terms of tests, specialists, and treatment. The next chapter discusses everything you need to know about the first trimester, for both the high-risk and routine pregnancy.

3

T1 Health
(Trimester 1)

If this is your first pregnancy, all of the changes in your body and the emotional investment you're putting into the pregnancy can be pretty overwhelming. In addition, you may feel worried, nervous, anxious, and ultimately terrified about the outcome of the pregnancy. If you've worked hard for the pregnancy after a long bout of delayed conception, your initial fears may revolve around losing the pregnancy—certainly not an unreasonable fear given the statistics. Or if you and your partner had no trouble getting pregnant, you might be thinking "It's all happening too fast—I'm not ready!"

This chapter is designed to address *all* of your concerns. To make your research as stress-free as possible, an alphabetical breakdown of symptoms is provided so you can access the information you need quickly. (Nothing is more maddening than having to read through a clump of symptoms that you're not experiencing!) You'll also find separate sections on morning sickness, nutrition, weight, and fitness. Finally, this chapter is packed with information on the stuff that anxiety dreams are made of: *things that can go wrong.* Bleeding and spotting, miscarriage, and ectopic pregnancy, as well as emergency procedures for those conditions. (Molar pregnancies are discussed in chapter 4, because they're usually diagnosed in the second trimester.) This information is included not to frighten you but *to empower* you, should you encounter these problems down the road.

How Does It Feel?

If you asked 10 different women how early pregnancy feels, you would get 10 completely different answers. It's important not to regard this section as an absolute, but rather as a general picture of the range of early pregnancy symptoms. You may experience some, all, or *none* of these symptoms. Some women may even find that they've "slept" through early pregnancy by not even realizing that they're pregnant until about the fourth month.

When we think about early pregnancy, most of us envision a woman with large, full breasts, hanging her head down into the toilet every morning as she vomits up her breakfast. Well, this really isn't an accurate picture for many women.

Pregnancy symptoms don't really appear until around week four. At this stage, you may notice a peculiar metallic taste in your mouth. By week five, your period may be either late or you may experience one or two scant periods. You may also feel as if you are about to get your period any minute. Your breasts will enlarge and begin to become tender. You may also feel bloated, stuffy, or headachy, all of which are symptoms attributed more often to PMS than pregnancy. Frequent urination is another major common symptom at this stage; however, it is also a symptom of urinary tract infections (UTIs), as discussed on page 78. Frequent urination during pregnancy is due to hormonal changes: Progesterone relaxes the muscles of the bladder and uterine wall.

By week six, your uterus will have grown to the size of a large orange, and your vagina will begin to change to a bluish color, which is due to an increased blood flow to the area. You may also begin to experience morning sickness by this point (if you are, in fact, destined to experience it at all). Morning sickness is discussed in detail on pages 81-83.

By week seven, you might experience some dizziness (discussed more on page 74). Little nodules (lumps) will appear on your breasts, and the aureola will darken as your nipples become more prominent.

By week eight, some foods might begin to make you sick—an extension of your morning sickness—and you may notice that your hair isn't as manageable as it used to be. You'll also notice a clear, whitish, odorless vaginal discharge, known as *leukorrhea,* which occurs due to hormonal changes.

By week nine, your skin changes, and wrinkles may be less obvious. Your gums may soften, which means that you'll need to stay on top of your dental hygiene program and perhaps floss more regularly. Meanwhile, your thyroid gland, discussed in chapter 2, will become more prominent. This is a *normal* part of pregnancy and should not be mistaken for a *goiter,* an enlarged thyroid gland that develops in people suffering from a thyroid disorder.

By week 10, your uterus has grown to the size of a grapefruit, and your breasts might be large enough to warrant a good support bra. It's possible to hear the fetal heartbeat with a Doppler stethoscope (an electronic stethoscope).

By week 11, if you are suffering from morning sickness, your nausea should begin to taper off, and although not immediately noticeable, your blood volume has increased considerably by this point. Nosebleeds are often a consequence of this, as discussed on page 77.

Finally, by week 12, the week that officially marks the end of the first trimester, you'll definitely need to have your first prenatal exam if you haven't been seen by a doctor yet. It is at *this* stage that your doctor will be able to feel your uterus with his or her fingers in an external exam because it has now risen *above* the pelvis.

The ABCs of Pregnancy

Now that you have a general idea of what symptoms make an appearance at various stages of this trimester, let's discuss them one by one. Because you won't be experiencing every conceivable first trimester symptom, I've organized this section alphabetically. That way, you can find information faster about the symptom affecting *you*.

Breast changes

Most women will feel changes in their breasts. The breasts will swell, tingle, throb, and/or hurt. This is because your breasts are developing milk glands. There is also an increased blood supply going to your breasts, so the veins will become more pronounced. Your nipples will also enlarge, become more erect, while your areola will darken and become broader. Some women will notice early on that their nipples are very sensitive and sore.

Constipation

During pregnancy, your bowel function slows down to ensure absorption of vitamins and nutrients from food. Progesterone also relaxes the smooth muscles of your small and large intestines. This slows down the entire digestive process, the result of which is constipation.

This is a nagging problem during pregnancy that tends to get worse as the pregnancy progresses. But rather than take laxatives, you should instead add more fiber to your diet; it's dangerous for your system to become dependent on laxatives. Adjust your diet to include more fruit, vegetables, fiber, and fluids, and less milk, calcium, and simple sugars. Try to enrich your diet with more fluids (about six to eight glasses per day), and try to eliminate particularly fatty foods. One to two tablespoons of unsulphured blackstrap molasses in warm water once or twice a day is a reliable old remedy for constipation. Molasses is also high in iron and trace minerals. And, of course, prune juice can often work miracles. Walking or mild physical exercise also helps get your bowels moving.

To make matters worse, you may also have hemorrhoids, which

will only aggravate constipation. Hemorrhoids are caused by hormonal changes and an enlarged uterus, which puts pressure on your pelvic veins. Because of this, try not to *force* your stools. If you'e on the toilet and nothing's happening, get up! If you sit there, strain, and force a bowel movement, you might either make your hemorrhoids worse or trigger an impending hemorrhoid. Get into the habit of waiting until the stools are "almost out" before you go to the bathroom.

Stool softeners, which can be prescribed by your doctor, might help. These will not work unless your fluid intake is high. Some doctors also suggest that you try sitting on the toilet for about 10 minutes after each meal. The stimulation of your stomach from eating will be transmitted right down through to your bowels, which may train your body to defecate at regular times each day. This is called the *gastro-colic reflex*. Finally, whatever you do—don't ignore the urge to defecate.

Dizziness

This is common, and is discussed under "Faintness" below.

Dyspnea (shortness of breath)

Nobody is really sure *why* shortness of breath occurs during this trimester. Some think that it's caused by increased levels of progesterone. Many women tend to think that dyspnea (pronounced disp-nee-ah) is weight-related, but this isn't the case at this stage because weight gain is usually fairly minimal. What doctors *do* know is that dyspnea can be a problem if you're asthmatic. In this case, consult your asthma specialist before you increase your asthma medication on your own. Otherwise, this symptom is nothing to worry about, but you should report it to your obstetrician nevertheless.

Emotional symptoms

The emotional symptoms of pregnancy vary greatly from woman to woman, but at this stage may mirror PMS mood swings. You may feel weepy, irritable, nervous, sad, or anxious. Some of these feelings have to do with the *social* impact of pregnancy; some of these feelings are attributed to major hormonal shifts in your body. Some foods, such as anything with caffiene, may be affecting you more powerfully than before the pregnancy. Fatigue, discussed next, also plays a role in your emotions by exaggerating certain feelings.

Your preparedness for the pregnancy will greatly affect your emotions as well. For example, if the pregnancy was unplanned and/or you don't have a strong emotional support system at home, you may suffer from more severe mood swings. If you've been planning the pregnancy and are excited about it, you may feel completely content and experience no significant emotional changes. If you feel that your emotional state is affecting how you function from day to day, you should seek counseling with a qualified social worker or therapist. You may just need to talk to someone, or you may benefit from speaking to other pregnant women who are experiencing similar feelings. Validation of your feelings is often the only medicine you need. Keep in mind, however, that if you have a history of psychiatric illness or clinical or major depression, your feelings may have more to do with your psychiatric state than your pregnancy. In other words, just because you're pregnant doesn't mean you're suddenly immune to the effects of a psychiatric illness. Depression is discussed in chapter 10.

Faintness

Feelings of faintness and dizziness are not unusual. The faintness happens because progesterone dilates the smooth muscle of the blood vessels and causes pooling of blood in the legs. In addition, a lot more blood begins to flow to the uterus. This can cause low blood pressure, which can result in fainting. Standing or sitting for long periods of time tends to trigger it. Doing exercises that get the blood circulating again can prevent this.

If you start to feel dizzy while you're standing, shifting your weight is also helpful. Lying flat on your back is often the worst thing you can do. The uterus can compress major arteries and cut off the blood supply to both you and your baby. Lying down this way can also cause your blood pressure to drop dangerously low. So, *lie on your side* if this is a problem. (This is usually more of a second trimester ailment.)

Faintness and dizziness can also be affected by poor eating habits. When your blood sugar is too low, you can develop a condition known as *hypoglycemia,* which is characterized by faintness and dizziness, irritability, shakiness, and headaches. Eating regularly will help prevent this, but eating *processed* foods will do you no good because the body tends to burn up chemically processed foods too quickly. The solution: eat fresh food at regular intervals.

Fatigue

Fatigue is a major symptom at this stage. This begins after the first missed period and persists until the 14th to 20th week of pregnancy. The remedy for this is simple: *Get more sleep!* Take naps in the afternoon if you're at home; nap after work if you're working through your pregnancy, and try to arrange for extra help around the house. About 10 hours of sleep a night is suggested during the first trimester. You'll probably need to adjust your schedule for this: Go to bed earlier than usual to get the rest you need and avoid going out if you feel too tired. Just use your common sense.

Headaches

Headaches are a common complaint during this trimester, but since no one really knows what causes headaches to begin with, nobody knows why they occur in pregnancy, either. Acetaminephen (Tylenol) appears to be safe for minor headaches and common aches and pains. If you're taking prescription medication for migraine headaches, make sure you check with your doctor before you use it. Don't take any other over-the-counter medications without consulting your doctor first. Some suggested natural remedies include putting a cool cloth on your head while lying down, eating frequently, and having your feet massaged (the big toe is apparently the acupressure site for the head).

Heartburn

As your uterus expands, it pushes the stomach up. Combine this with a slower digestive system (see "Constipation" above) and the result is heartburn. Try eliminating liquids with meals, which will cause you to eat more slowly and improve your digestion. Avoid antacids with sodium bicarbonates. Heartburn is discussed more in chapter 4, as it tends to be more of a second- and third-trimester issue.

Hemorrhoids

Unfortunately, few pregnant women can avoid these miserable things. Hemorrhoids are swollen veins around the anus. They're caused by an expanding uterus, which puts more pressure on the area, as well as an increase in blood volume. Progesterone also slows down your circulation to accommodate your growing uterus. And constipation can further aggravate the situation. Hemorrhoids will usually develop in the rectum, but sometimes they can develop in the vagina, making intercourse very uncomfortable. Sitting and standing for long periods of time can also aggravate hemorrhoids. There are hemorrhoid medications (such as Preparation H) that you can take with your doctor's permission to relieve the pain. Warm baths are also helpful, and frequently shifting your positions from standing to sitting can help. Also see "Constipation" above.

Insomnia

If you're a coffee drinker, you might suffer bouts of insomnia in early pregnancy. Avoid caffeine in this case. Otherwise, anxiousness about the pregnancy, or other symptoms (like hemorrhoids!) may be keeping you up at night. There's not much you can do about this other than ride it out. Do not take any sleeping medications!

Menstrual cycle changes

Obviously, you won't be menstruating regularly, but you might continue to bleed very scantily throughout this trimester. In fact, women often don't realize they're pregnant until about three months into the pregnancy because of this. Whether you have bled scantily or have missed your period, you may, as discussed above, feel a range of premenstrual symptoms: bloating, breast tenderness, headaches, and so on. Many women will dismiss the possibility of pregnancy because of this.

Although period changes usually won't be noticed until about weeks 4 and 5, you can spot as early as seven days after conception. This is known as *implantation bleeding* and is normal vaginal spotting caused by the formation of new blood vessels, *but* it's rarely experienced.

If you've been using a basal body thermometer, you might also notice a slight rise in your temperature. Normally, your temperature rises about one degree during ovulation. But if you're charting your temperature and notice that this increase remains beyond ten days, it's a sign that you may be pregnant.

Morning sickness (nausea)

See the separate section on morning sickness on page 81-83. This is very common.

Nosebleeds

The increased blood supply in your body during preganacy strains the veins in your nose. To treat nosebleeds, pinch your nostrils together, sit up, apply pressure for five minutes, then put a cold cloth on the back of your neck. Nosebleeds are usually nothing to worry about, but if you're prone to high blood pressure or have a pre-existing hypertension condition, make sure you report your nosebleeds to your doctor. He or she will need to monitor your blood pressure and make sure that the nosebleeds aren't a symptom of hypertension.

Numbness

Your expanding uterus can put pressure on your nerves, which sometimes causes numbness and tingling. This usually isn't anything to worry about. In the second and third trimesters, water retention can put pressure on the median nerve in your wrist, cutting off feeling in your hand and fingers. This is called *carpal tunnel syndrome*, which is discussed in chapter 4. If you're diabetic, report any feelings of numbness to your doctor immediately. This could be a sign that your diabetes is out of control.

Urinary frequency

Why do all pregnant women urinate more frequently? First, your uterus is enlarging and pressing down on your bladder. Second, since you're retaining more water, you have more that needs to be eliminated. If you experience burning or a poor stream when you do urinate, you may be suffering from a *urinary tract infection,* a separate problem that is, unfortunately, common during pregnancy. See the next section for more details.

Urinary tract infections (UTIs)

UTIs are very common during pregnancy. They are usually caused by the bacteria *Escherichia coli,* which travel from the colon through the urethra to the bladder. The most common UTI is *cystitis,* which is either an inflammation or infection of the bladder. A classic symptom of cystitis is a painful or burning sensation in the urethra (known as *dysuria,* meaning painful urination). Many women with cystitis also constantly feel like they have to urinate (some women report that they have to urinate up to 60 times a day), but find that almost nothing comes out when they *do* try. Other symptoms of UTIs may include blood in the urine, known as *hematuria,* or pus in the urine, known as *pyuria.* Even severe cystitis is usually more painful than serious—and can be treated with antibiotics safe for use during pregnancy.

Sometimes cystitis clears up on its own within about 24 hours, but don't wait around for this to happen. See your doctor ASAP if you notice any symptoms so you can be treated ASAP! If your symptoms are straightforward, many doctors will treat you without culturing, but it's important to rule out a vaginal infection *first.* In this case, the burning would occur because the urine is irritating a *vaginal* inflammation. In fact, it's common for women to think they have a UTI when they really have *vaginitis,* or an inflammation of the vagina. Vaginitis is often the result of a *yeast* infection (discussed below), which is also common in pregnancy.

For a simple case of cystitis, you'll be prescribed *nitrofuranetoine* (macrodentin, macrobid), *ampicillin* (Ampicin), *amoxicillin* (Amoxil), or *trimethoprine/sulfamethoxazole TMP/SXT* (Septra). Septra should be avoided in later pregnancy. You'll then need to give another urine sample to make sure the infection has cleared up. You'll need to take these antibiotics for about 10 to 14 days. A follow-up urine culture will also need to be taken. For more information on UTIs, check out *The Gynecological Sourcebook*, listed in Appendix B at the back of this book.

Vaginal changes

As the blood flow increases to your uterus, your vagina may turn a bluish color. You will also notice the leukorrhea (white, clear, odorless, and mucusy discharge) discussed earlier. If, however, there is an odor to the discharge, or itchiness, you most likely have a vaginal infection, the most common of which is yeast. (Yeast infections are discussed next.)

Some women also may notice shooting pains in the vagina, which is caused by uterine pressure on the nerve endings. This pain is fleeting and isn't anything to worry about. In any case, there is not much you can do about it other than ride it out.

Yeast infections

Yeast infections are caused by *candida albicans,* a type of fungus that belongs to the plant kingdom. It is a "friendly" fungus. Under normal circumstances, candida is always in your vagina, mouth, and digestive tract. For a variety of reasons, candida can overgrow and reproduce too much of itself, changing from a harmless one-cell fungus into long branches of yeast cells called *mycelia*. This is known as *candidiasis* (pronounced candid-eye-isis).

Generally, any changes to your vagina's normal acidic environment can make you vulnerable to yeast infections. The list of factors that can affect your vaginal environment is actually quite long, but the most common factor is pregnancy. Pregnancy makes the vagina less acidic and increases the amount of sugar stored in the vaginal cell walls. And yeast *love* sugar! Diabetic women also suffer from chronic yeast infections because of their blood sugar levels. (Sometimes the first sign of diabetes is a stubborn vaginal yeast infection, so if you suffer from chronic yeast infections, get screened for diabetes.) If you're pregnant *and* diabetic, you'll probably be plagued by yeast infections throughout your pregnancy.

Anything that interferes with the immune system will also make yeast thrive. For example, antibiotics not only kill harmful bacteria, but also often kill the friendly bacteria that are in the vagina, to fend off infection. So if your doctor prescribes antibiotics for, let's say, cystitis, ask him or her about what to do to prevent a yeast infection.

Severe itching and a curdlike or cottage-cheesy discharge are classic symptoms of a vaginal yeast infection. The discharge, interestingly, may smell like baking bread, fermenting yeast, or even brewing beer. Other symptoms are swelling, redness, and irritation of the outer and inner vaginal lips; painful sex; and painful urination due to an irritation of the urethra. Women who have candidiasis are usually *not* asymptomatic.

Vaginal yeast infections are so common that, in the United States, over-the-counter medications such as *miconazole* (Monistat), *nystatin* (Mycostatin and many others), and even an herbal product, *Yeaststat*, are readily available. *But don't ever self-medicate without consulting your doctor and confirming that what you have is indeed yeast.* Generally, all over-the-counter vaginal yeast medications are antifungal creams, suppositories, or oral antifungals. There are numerous brands available, and your doctor will recommend one that's safe to use during pregnancy. A doctor will confirm a yeast infection by taking a vaginal swab, also known as a "wet prep."

There are some natural remedies that will treat the symptoms of yeast infections, but will not cure the infection. Among these is eating two small containers of plain yogurt with active yogurt culture daily. For unbearable itching, 1% hydrocotisone cream (available in the U.S. over the counter) is helpful.

There *are* preventative measures you can take to ward off yeast infections during your pregnancy, including the following.

- *Don't wear tight clothing around your vagina.* Since you won't need maternity clothing just yet, you'll probably be wearing much of your usual wardrobe. Unfortunately, this can spell trouble for your vagina. Tight pants, panties, and nylon pantyhose prevent your vagina from "breathing" and make it a warmer and moister environment for yeast. Wear looser pants that allow your vagina to breathe, switch to knee-highs or old-fashioned stockings, and wear pantyhose only on special occasions. Also go "bottomless" to bed to let air into your vagina.

- *Wear only 100%-cotton clothing and/or natural fibers around your vagina.* Wearing synthetic underwear and polyester pants is not a good idea. All-cotton underwear and denim, wool, or rayon pants that are loose fitting are fine.

- *Watch your toilet habits.* Always wipe from front to back with toilet paper. Otherwise you can introduce rectal waste into your vagina. After a looser bowel movement, wet the toilet paper and clean your rectal area thoroughly so that fecal material doesnt stay on your underwear and wind up in your vagina. To prepare for less hygienic circumstances, carry some baby wipes with you.

- *Don't insert anything into a dry vagina.* Whether it's a penis or a sex toy, make sure your vagina is well lubricated before insertion. Dry vaginas can be prone to abrasions during insertion, which make an excellent home for yeast.

- *Avoid long car trips on vinyl seats.* New research indicates that vinyl seats increase a woman's risk of developing a yeast infection because the vinyl traps moisture and doesn't allow the crotch area to breathe.

Morning Sickness

Morning sickness is the infamous nausea and vomiting women tend to experience during early pregnancy. Between 60 and 80% of all women suffer from morning sickness in their first trimester. Be forewarned: Morning sickness may *begin* in the morning, but it often persists 24 hours a day for the first few weeks of pregnancy. Sometimes the nausea isn't bad enough to cause vomiting but is just sort of ever-present, warded off by eating dry crackers or drinking juice.

In more severe cases of morning sickness, the nausea and vomiting begins between six and eight weeks after your last menstrual period, persists strongly until about 14 weeks after your last period, and then either disappears or gets much better. However, it can persist well into the second trimester, too, and can even last the duration of the pregnancy. While most doctors and pregnancy books tell you that morning sickness lasts for about 12 weeks, the average length is more like 17 weeks.

There are also numerous other symptoms that accompany morning sickness. These include an aversion to certain tastes or smells that never bothered you before, such as coffee, cigarette smoke, meat, and my favorite example (from a chronic dieter), salad! Sometimes just the sight of some of these foods may send you heaving. Some women find it difficult to prepare any foods and may be turned off every food except one in particular, such as grapefruit, yogurt, or crackers.

Skipping meals and fasting is the worst thing you can do. Child-bearing practitioners suggest eating frequent, small meals or snacks. Nibbling on dry crackers continuously throughout the day and keeping cracker stashes at the office, your bedside, and in the car really helps. The nausea is caused by changes in hormone levels that affect your stomach lining and stomach acids, so an empty stomach tends to aggravate the nausea. Giving your stomach something to actually *digest* is the best way to combat it. There is also a strong connection between nausea and low blood sugar levels. If you're diabetic, this could mean trouble, so make sure you stay on top of your blood sugar levels. The cracker stashes also will help prevent hypoglycemia.

One interesting theory about the causes of morning sickness is that the nausea in early pregnancy is a self-defense mechanism; you're expelling toxins from your body that may harm the fetus. The idea is that, if certain foods are bad for the fetus, you are protecting it by either vomiting them up or being repulsed by their tastes or smells. This theory is based on research that indicates that women with little or no nausea and vomiting are *two to three times* more likely to miscarry, presumably because they are eating foods that are harming the embryo. Statistics also show that women with morning sickness tend to have more favorable outcomes than women who don't have it. But if you're *not* nauseous, don't worry about it!

Many practitioners recommend that women experiencing morning sickness should eat whatever they are craving, be it ice cream or potato chips. Although fresh, healthy food is always better, if you're vomiting everything up, eating whatever you can keep down is the best.

The problem with nonstop nausea and vomiting is that you might become malnourished or dehydrated. Try to sip fluids such as fruit juices, and remember to keep drinking water. (You don't have to worry about drinking milk just yet, which is even nauseating to many women who aren't pregnant!) If you're vomiting more than three times a day, see your doctor and make sure that you're not dehydrated. Most women have enough reserves in their body to nourish the fetus regardless of how nauseated they are.

Is there anything you can do to *prevent* morning sickness? Perhaps. It has been shown that taking a vitamin B6 supplement is effective in reducing severe morning sickness in pregnancy, but it doesn't seem to have any effect on mild and moderate nausea.

In another study, Hungarian researchers divided women into three groups: Prior to conception and throughout the first trimester, one group took multivitamin supplements, the second group took multimineral supplements, while the last group was given placebos. The intent of the study was to prove whether taking vitamins can reduce the risk of neural tube birth defects. But the study wound up shedding far more light on morning sickness than birth defects! Apparently the women on the placebo reported vertigo, nausea, and vomiting serious enough to seek treatment much more than those women taking vitamins and minerals. So you may be able to ward off your nausea by taking vitamin pills! Check out this option with your doctor!

A final word: Just because you're in early pregnancy, it doesn't mean you don't have a stomach flu or another ailment causing the nausea. So be sure to check it out if the nausea persists beyond what's tolerable.

Multiple-Pregnancy Symptoms

Early pregnancy symptoms for women carrying multiple fetuses will be more noticeable and severe than those of women carrying one fetus. Instead of fatigued, you may feel utterly exhausted; you'll gain more weight than single-fetus carriers (weight is discussed more fully below); and you may suffer from insomnia, more severe backaches, hemorrhoids, edema, and *very* severe morning sickness. You may experience anemia, as more than one fetus will demand more iron than you're capable of producing. You may also notice numbness and pain around your upper ribs and breastbone, which is caused by a more rapid expansion of your uterus. The pressure on the stomach created by more than one baby will also prevent you from being able to eat large meals. You'll need to eat about six small meals a day, and should work out a food plan with your doctor or a qualified nutritionist. You'll also need to be on vitamin supplements, such as iron and vitamin B.

In general, since multiple-birth pregnancies may not be detected until the second trimester, it's important to take note of more severe symptoms and tell your doctor that you suspect you may be carrying multiple fetuses. Carrying multiple fetuses is a high-risk pregnancy, and you'll need to be under the care of a perinatologist or experienced obstetrician in this case. Women who are more likely to have twins are: pregnant as a result of fertility drugs; black; or those who have a family history of twins or multiple-birth pregnancies.

Nutrition Concerns

Eating well is important during your pregnancy. The best thing to do is request a referral to a *nutritionist,* and work out your daily nutritional needs with him or her. Or, book a separate appointment with either your doctor or midwife to design an appropriate diet that's right for you. The following nutritional information is intended as a *general* guideline only. Not every pregnancy is standard. Each woman experiences different symptoms, has a different medical history, and lives a different lifestyle, and, therefore, *needs to eat different things.* Some women will need to take a vitamin supplement, while other women will need to avoid vitamin supplements to relieve or prevent other symptoms.

One of the major problems with the current nutritional information on pregnancy is that *there's too much of it!* Many diet plans are too overwhelming and puritanical for the average, working, nauseous, stressed-out pregnant woman to follow. One woman I interviewed was relieved to discover from her doctor that she could have one cup of real coffee each morning. She had read that caffeine in any amount would cause fetal abnormalities. Her doctor felt that, in light of the fact that this woman was working, battling traffic jams, and fighting off fatigue, one cup of coffee each morning was appropriate for *her.* On the other hand, someone else more sensitive to caffeine may not be able to have coffee.

Another concern is the "no junk food" rule. Pregnant women in the 1990s are only human. Eating a Big Mac, a chocolate bar, or a bag of potato chips once in a while is *not* going to cause fetal abnormalities. If you're caught in a horrendous traffic jam, eating *something*—even if it's not a sandwich made with all-natural, free-range chicken—is better than nothing. Furthermore, many workplaces aren't exactly pregnant-friendly. You might be busy all day and have time only for fast food, which you can always adjust to your needs. (Even McDonalds has salads!)

As for all that milk! What if you have a lactose intolerance problem and don't feel like taking Lactaid all the time? What if you have other food allergies? What if you're a vegetarian (and eat neither dairy nor eggs)? What if you're diabetic? What if you're anemic or are on certain medications that interfere with some foods? Weight gain is also highly individualized. What if you're battling a weight problem already? What if you have a history of eating disorders?

The bottom line is that nutrition during pregnancy is *too important* to get out of a book or a magazine article. Your age, weight, history, and pregnancy symptoms will *all* affect your diet and vitamin supplementation during pregnancy. Besides, your diet may need to continuously change throughout your pregnancy.

The *General* Guidelines

Nutritional experts will tell you that you should prepare to weigh somewhere between 20 and 30 pounds more by the time you deliver (based on a woman of average height in good health). If you break this estimated weight gain down week by week, you should be one to two pounds heavier by week 10, which translates into consuming an extra 300 calories per day for a total of about 2,600 calories per day. Very few pregnancies reflect this even amount of calories.

What will these extra calories consist of? More protein and calcium, and a balanced mixture of minerals and vitamins, including iron and folic acid supplements. Here's what one plan recommends for your daily diet: four 8-ounce cups of milk or dairy products (you can substitute yogurt and cheese for milk); four servings of protein (fish, poultry, lean beef, beans, peas, lentils, peanut butter, or nuts); two servings of leafy greens; one serving of fresh fruit and vegetables high in vitamin C (don't forget that a plain baked potato is an excellent source of vitamin C); one serving of a deep yellow or orange fruit; four servings of grains (bread, pasta, muffin, cereals, rice); and 8 to 10 cups of fluids a day (it does not have to be milk).

Why do you need to eat all of this food? Protein is critical for the growth of fetal tissue and may prevent toxemia from developing (discussed in chapter 2). Vitamins A, D, E, and K, present in dairy and eggs, are important for the growth of fetal tissue. The fiber in leafy greens, grains, and fruits is important for regularity. Two kinds of carbohydrates also are important: complex (starches) and simple (sugars, which are found in fruits, vegetables, and whole grains). The glucose from simple carbohydrates helps fight fatigue in pregnancy and helps burn fat more efficiently. A diet too low in carbohydrates can lead to the creation of toxic ketones in the blood, which can create fatty acids harmful to the fetus.

Because the fetus is taking calcium from your bones and teeth, you'll need to replace the calcium you're losing by taking in about 50 percent more than normal (about 1200 mg. of calcium per day). This will also help prevent osteoporosis (bone loss) from occurring after menopause. High sources of calcium include dairy products, sardines, salmon, oysters, shrimp, tofu, kale, and broccoli. These foods are also high sources of phosphorus, which is necessary to absorb calcium.

Iron is needed for the production of red blood cells, which carry oxygen to your tissues and to the fetus. During pregnancy, the blood volume in your body doubles, which doubles your iron requirements, The fetus will take iron from you whether you can spare it or not, so to prevent anemia, you'll need a daily iron supplement of roughly 20 mg. Eating foods high in vitamin C, folic acid, and vitamin B_{12} will help you absorb iron efficiently from the other foods in your diet .

Iodine and chromium are necessary to strengthen your bones and the fetus's skeleton. Iodine is found in iodized salt and shellfish; chromium is found in whole-grain breads and cereals.

Zinc is needed to strengthen the enzymes that drive your metabolism. Roughly 20 mg. of zinc are needed during pregnancy, and that amount can be cut in half when you're breastfeeding. You'll find zinc in almonds, eggs, peanuts, beef, walnuts, liver, herring, and oysters.

All the B vitamins can be found in lean meats, whole grains, liver, seeds, nuts, wheat germ, and dairy products. The most important are B_6 and folic acid. Normally, you'd need about 2.5 mg, but when you're pregnant, you require more like 10 mg each day. The best way to get what you need is through a supplement prescribed by your doctor or nutritionist.

Vitamin A, which is found in orange and yellow fruits and vegetables and in dairy products, is important for the development of the baby's thyroid gland, future tooth enamel, and hair. *You* need vitamin A for healthy skin and mucous membranes, such as those in your vagina, which will come in handy during labor! Too much vitamin A can be damaging, however, so make sure you consult a nutritionist before overdosing on yams.

Vitamin D is manufactured by the sun and is necessary for the absorption of calcium. It's found in milk, but you can also get it from exposure to the sun or by taking a supplement. Again, too much is dangerous, so consult a nutritionist for the proper dosage.

Vitamin E helps your baby's lungs mature. It's found in vegetable oils, wheat germ, soybeans, broccoli, brussels sprouts, whole grains, and eggs.

One good way of combining all of these dizzying lists of vitamins and nutrients is to make soups. For example, to beef up your calcium, fiber, and fluid intake, you could make cream of spinach soup (a snap with a food processor), getting all these nutrients in one bang. The point is, get creative. Make carrot pancakes, almond butter sandwiches, or anything you like! You get the idea.

Special circumstances

Again, while every pregnancy is unique when it comes to dietary requirements, the following groups of women will *absolutely* need a nutritionist:

- *Women carrying multiple fetuses.* You'll need a lot more calories and nutrients!
- *Pregnant adolescents.* You're still growing and need more nutrients (particularly calcium) than adults.
- *Women with pregnancies close together.* Your "supplies" may be depleted, so you'll need extra calories and nutrients.
- *Vegetarians.* You'll need extra vitamin B_{12} and will need to combine various groups of proteins. You'll also need more calories, dairy, and eggs.
- *Women with food and/or milk allergies.* You'll need more *options,* which a nutritionist can provide.
- *Women with eating disorders.* You may have trouble accepting your new body and food requirements. Please consult a nutritionist and possibly a therapist for the best outcome.

Things you probably already know . . .

- Don't take any medications unless your doctor prescribes them.
- Try to avoid or cut down on caffeine. Not only is it associated with late first-term and second-term miscarriages and low birthweights, it's a diuretic, which causes you to urinate more and *lose calcium.* It also tends to restrict the oxygen flow to the

uterus and may enter the fetal blood stream. (You don't want your newborn craving Folger's just yet!)

- Artificial sweetners such as Aspartame are *technically* considered safe, but doctors will still tell you not to use them. And you probably shouldn't.

- Smoking is *always* a bad idea, especially when you're pregnant. Smoking during pregnancy can lead to the premature rupture of membranes, premature birth, perinatal death, placental abnormalities, and bleeding during pregnancy. Respiratory illnesses are more common in children born to smokers.

- Regarding the drinking of alcoholic beverages, *no safe amount of alcohol in pregnancy has ever been determined.* Fetal alcohol syndrome is associated with *heavy* alcohol use during pregnancy (as opposed to one glass of wine per trimester), and can cause mental and physical retardation, strange facial characteristics, and low birthweights in babies. Even the Old Testament warns: "Behold, thou shalt conceive, and bear a son, and now drink no wine or strong drink." In ancient Rome, alcohol was forbidden on the wedding night because its effects on conception were feared. And, in 1736, the College of Physicians in London, England, reported that alcohol during pregnancy caused "weak, feeble and distempered children." Currently, 1.9 of each 1,000 babies is estimated to be born with fetal alcohol syndrome, which is considered a major cause of mental retardation worldwide.

- Marijuana, cocaine, amphetamines, and other narcotics are bad news, and even worse news in pregnancy. All of these drugs are associated with preterm delivery, low birthweight, sudden onset of uterine contractions and placental abruption (cocaine), stillbirths, birth defects, addicted newborns, sudden infant death syndrome, and many more nightmarish consequences.

Things you may not know . . .
- Some herbs can be very harmful during pregnancy. Consult your doctor before you start taking herbal remedies for any reason.

- Aspirin is *not* okay and can do a lot of damage. Don't take it unless your doctor prescribes it.

A Word About Weight

Yes, you're technically "eating for two," but remember that your fetus will seldom grow to weigh over 10 pounds. You'll need to work out a realistic food plan and weight-gain strategy with your nutritionist. Don't look at your pregnancy as a food-bingeing free for all. Gaining too much weight will make it more difficult for you to take it off after the delivery and may also aggravate other problems down the road.

By the time you begin the second trimester, you only need to have gained an average 2 to 6 pounds. Assuming that by your delivery date you will weigh between 20 and 30 pounds heavier, here's the way this average weight gain is compiled: Your baby will weigh about 7.5 pounds, the placenta weighs about 1 pound, the amniotic fluid about 2 pounds, the uterus about 2.5 pounds, breast tissue about 3 pounds, increased blood volume adds about 4 pounds, and your maternal fat stores weigh between 4 and 8 pounds. That gives you a total ranging between 24 and 28 pounds; if the baby weighs in larger, you'll be up to at least 30 pounds.

Again, all of this weight-gain information is based on the average pregnancy of a woman of average size. The bottom line is that you should gain the right amount of weight for *you* to ensure the health of your baby. If you're underweight to begin with, you'll need to start gaining weight while you try to conceive. If you're overweight, try to lose some weight prior to conception, but *never* diet during the pregnancy.

Fitness and Exercise

Both fitness and exercise are important, but in moderation. Your doctor or midwife is the best judge of what kind of activities are appropriate. Some women will need to speed up their activities and become more fit, while others will need to slow down. There are several good aerobics classes designed for pregnant women that work the right muscles, and prevent you from overdoing it. Whatever you decide, it's best to exercise under the supervision of a trained aerobics or fitness instructor.

One benefit to getting in shape during pregnancy is that you'll be more prepared for the physical work involved with labor. In general, the better shape you're in, the easier labor will be. But if you're too active, it could keep you from gaining enough weight for a healthy pregnancy. You should avoid any contact sport where your abdominal area could be hit or bumped and any activities where you could fall, such as bicycling. Swimming is probably one of the best exercises during pregnancy; it helps reduce edema, is relaxing, and won't harm the fetus or injure you in any way.

Things that Can Go Wrong

When something goes wrong at this stage, it generally has to do with the pregnancy's not taking. This usually means two things: a miscarriage (bleeding and cramping are the main symptoms) or an ectopic pregnancy (sharp, abdominal cramping or searing pain on one side, depending on the tube). Some women don't even *realize* they're pregnant until they experience one of these common first-trimester problems.

Ectopic pregnancies were considered a less common occurrence until about five years ago, when the results of sexually transmitted diseases (STDs), pelvic inflammatory disease (PID), and assisted conception started to factor into the childbearing population. If you've had PID (well over one million North American women do), you are at a higher risk of suffering an ectopic pregnancy. If you're walking around with undiagnosed chlamydia or gonorrhea, you're also at risk for this. *Some studies estimate that as many as 50% of all women between the ages of 18 and 30 have chlamydia and don't know it.* This is why it's important to be regularly screened for STDs, as stressed in chapters 1 and 2.

As for miscarriage, one in six pregnancies ends in miscarriage, *and 75% of these miscarriages occur before 12 weeks.* The risk of a miscarriage also increases with age. This is why it's crucial to have your birthing team and birthing facility in place *now* (see chapter 1).

While the majority of women *will* carry full-term, it is the women who *don't* who typically need more information. This is why I've provided "Things that Can Go Wrong" sections in this chapter, as well as in chapters 4 and 6.

Bleeding

Bleeding during pregnancy isn't normal, but it's not *unusual,* either. Nor does it mean that a miscarriage is imminent. Some women may continue to have scant bleeding during this trimester or may experience the implantation bleeding discussed earlier in this chapter. Vaginal bleeding can also occur if you have an infection of some kind, a polyp, or a fibroid. It's always important to note whether any pain accompanies your staining or bleeding: Staining or bleeding with no pain is better news than staining or bleeding accompanied by cramps. However, bleeding or spotting of *any* kind should be reported immediately to avoid any risk.

The most dangerous kind of bleeding at this point is heavy bleeding, which is when you need to change sanitary pads about every hour. Other danger signs to watch out for are *other symptoms* accompanying the bleeding, such as cramps, pain in the abdomen, fever, weakness, or vomiting. If the blood has clumps of tissue in it, this is also a bad sign. In this case, save your pad, stick it in a baggie—clumps and all—and take it to the doctor to look at. The clumps may provide important clues to what's going on. You may also notice an unusual odor. If light bleeding or spotting continues for more than three days, this is another, less obvious danger sign.

Regardless of why you're bleeding, you'll need to follow the emergency procedures outlined at the end of this chapter. You'll then need to undergo certain tests, including an internal pelvic exam, a blood test to see if your level of hCG (human chorionic gonadotropin) is normal, and an ultrasound.

Miscarriage

There are several reasons why a miscarriage occurs. Several studies indicate that about 60% of all first-time, first-trimester miscarriages occur because of genetic abnormalities. It's your body's way of doing its own genetic engineering, expelling malformed fetuses. More than 90% of women who miscarry once will go on to have successful pregnancies.

As far as I'm concerned, a first-trimester miscarriage is very much a *pregnancy* issue, not an infertility issue. It's important for all women in their first trimester to learn about miscarriage so they don't panic needlessly and can be prepared in the event that it happens.

Symptoms

Heavy bleeding and cramping anywhere between the end of the second month to the end of the third month are classic signs that you're in the process of miscarrying. Cramps without any bleeding are also a danger sign that you're miscarrying. The bleeding can be heavy enough to soak several pads in an hour, or may be "manageable" and more like a heavy period. You may also be experiencing *unbearable* cramping that renders you incapacitated. Sometimes you can "pass clots," which are dark red clumps that look like small pieces of raw beef liver, or you may pass grayish or pink tissue. A miscarriage can also be taking place at this stage if you have persistent, light bleeding and more mild cramping.

If you suspect a miscarriage . . .

In the United States, if you're under the care of a private physician, you will usually have a chance to consult with your doctor about your symptoms over the phone (most of them have 24-hour pagers). Depending on your situation, your doctor may be able to evaluate your problem over the phone; ask you to come into his or her office for an ultrasound, which can determine the status of the fetus; or ask you to meet him/her at the hospital. If you *are* miscarrying, a D & C (dilation and curettage) procedure can be scheduled at a convenient time for you rather than done as an "emergency" procedure. In fact, many doctors in private practice can actually do a better job of evaluating the problem in their offices than doctors in a hospital emergency room, who, of course, wouldn't be as familiar with your history as your own doctor.

If you're an American woman in a less-exclusive healthcare plan, or a Canadian woman (Canadian physicians do not have appropriate ultrasound equipment in their offices), you will need to inform your doctor's office of your symptoms and *go directly to the birthing facility*. Ask for either or both your midwife and/or your doctor to *meet* you there. Someone will take care of you when you get to the birthing facility. (Even if it's not a hospital, all birthing centers are staffed for emergencies.) Once you're in the hospital, your doctor will be able to tell whether you're miscarrying and, if so, what stage the miscarriage is in. He or she will do a pelvic exam and/or ultrasound. You might be sent home to wait it out, which is often the only thing to do. Sometimes it takes several hours for a miscarriage to run its course. Or, depending on what's going on, you might need to stay and have an emergency D & C procedure.

When you miscarry before 20 weeks, it's called a *spontaneous abortion*. However, there are several kinds of spontaneous abortions. Whether you stay in the hospital or are sent home will depend on what kind of miscarriage you're experiencing.

- *Threatened abortion.* Your cervix is still closed and holding everything in securely, but you're having cramps and bleeding or staining. Your doctor will examine you and check the fetal heartbeat. You may also need an ultrasound. Then you'll be ordered to bed. In some cases, the bleeding will stop and the pregnancy will continue normally. In other cases, you might miscarry anyway because of unsalvageable problems, such as severe genetic deformities.
- *Inevitable abortion.* In this case, nature has already taken its course and the process of miscarriage has started. Bleeding is heavy, cramps increase, and the cervix begins to dilate. You may wind up expelling everything while it's still intact: the fetus, amniotic sac, and placenta, accompanied by a lot of blood. This is the most traumatic kind of first-trimester mis-

carriage because you'll need to save what you've just expelled in case your doctor wants to perform tests. Sometimes you'll have to dig these things out of the toilet. If you're going through this, try not to be alone. Call a friend or make sure your partner is with you. If your doctor suspects an *inevitable abortion,* abnormal bleeding is usually heavy enough to warrant a D & C before any tissue passes out on its own. However, if a D & C is not done, the pregnancy tissue would come out on its own eventually. Your doctor may want to perform tests on the tissue. But in general, it's difficult to determine the cause of an abortion by examining or testing expelled tissue.

- *Incomplete abortion.* This is when some, but not all, pregnancy tissue has been spontaneously expelled. Usually what remains is fragments of the placenta. This needs to be corrected with a D & C procedure, which will clean out the uterus and help it to heal. You'll still need to save whatever comes out, which will look like clumpy pieces of blood.

- *Complete abortion.* This is when all pregnancy tissue is passed spontaneously. You will be sent home and will *slowly* expel everything by steadily bleeding. This will feel like a miserable period, but everything will come out in time. Sometimes an ultrasound may help determine if there's anything left that might require a D&C. The bleeding can actually go on for days until you're finally done. In this case, save anything that looks like pregnancy tissue and show it to your doctor.

- *Missed abortion.* This is also very traumatic. The fetus dies in the uterus but doesn't come out. You may not have symptoms that anything is wrong for quite some time. This is when you just lightly spot. In this situation, all of your pregnancy symptoms will gradually disappear, and you obviously wont progress at all. This condition is frequently diagnosed during a routine exam, and the fetal heartbeat can no longer be heard. Treatment depends on the duration of the pregnancy.

What are the odds?

The risk of miscarriage increases with age. The risk is about 10% for women in their 20s, and skyrockets to 50% for women in their mid-40s. This means that a significant portion of thirty-something pregnancies will end this way. There are all kinds of reasons why you might be miscarrying, but 90% of all women who miscarry either once or twice do go on to have normal pregnancies and deliveries. Usually, the reason has to do with a fetus's "self-terminating" because it wasn't developing properly. You'll need to wait anywhere from three to six months after a miscarriage before you try again. Choose an appropriate barrier method to prevent conception during this period.

One cause of miscarriage has to do with untreated bacterial infections, such as mycoplasma. If left untreated, mycoplasma can lead to an inflamed endometrium (endometritis), which can interfere with the embryo implanting. Another cause of some miscarriages is the effect of certain toxins that include anesthetic gases. Exposure to lead and mercury are also causes, but usually these toxins are discovered before a *second* miscarriage.Other causes cited for repeated miscarriage include genetic problems, structural problems involving the uterus or cervix (such as an incompetent cervix), luteal phase defects, and thyroid disease (if it's not treated promptly).

After two consecutive miscarriages, you should *stop* trying and go for diagnostic tests to see *why* you're miscarrying. Often, the reasons are unknown and you'll go on to have a successful third pregnancy. In fact, even after two miscarriages, there's a 70% chance that your third pregnancy will be fine. But if a reason does turn up, it may be easy to fix, and finding the cause at this point will prevent further trauma to you. Possible causes of miscarriage at this stage involve hormonal deficiencies that interfere with fetal development, uterine structural problems, genetic error, and blood incompatibility.

When miscarriages keep repeating (three or more in a row), this is considered an *infertility* problem. *However, one or two miscarriages do not make you infertile and are generally not precursors to future problems.*

Some women may have more severe reactions to pregnancy loss

than others. These reactions may include sleep disturbances, psychosomatic illness, worsening of a previous illness (such as asthma), irritability, and avoiding social contact (particularly friends with children or friends who are pregnant). A good therapist can help you work through some of these feelings, which are valid and common under these circumstances.

It's also helpful to seek out other women who have gone through pregnancy loss as well. There are several support groups for women who have miscarried once or twice. For more information on pregnancy loss and miscarriage, review the resources, organized alphabetically by subject at the back of this book.

Repeated miscarriage

If you've miscarried more than twice in a row prior to 20 weeks, you're prone to what's known in lay terminology as "repeated miscarriages." (Clinical terms for this are *habitual abortion* or *recurrent fetal loss*.)

If you have no history of full-term pregnancies, then you suffer from *primary repeated miscarriage*. If you've had one child or even a stillbirth at term, you have *secondary repeated miscarriage*. In most cases of repeated miscarriage, the cause is found; in a few cases, nothing is ever discovered as the definitive cause. Women who have suffered as many as six or seven miscarriages, however, can go on to have a successful pregnancy.

Some doctors believe that a significant number of repeated first-trimester miscarriages are caused by a progesterone deficiency; others don't subscribe to this theory at all, even though there is strong evidence to support it.

Once your ovary spits out a follicle, the empty shell turns into a corpus luteum. If you imagine a single pea pod, the pea is the follicle which will become the egg, while the pod is what will turn into a corpus luteum, which should produce progesterone once the embryo implants. Human chorionic gonadotropin (HCG), secreted from the developing placenta, stimulates the corpus luteum to make progesterone. As the placenta matures at about 7 weeks, it takes over progesterone production. However, if the corpus luteum is not functioning properly and is therefore not making adequate amounts of progesterone, you will miscarry. Hormonal tests that include an endometrial biopsy will confirm whether you have this type of luteal phase defect.

The treatment is simple, involving daily dosages of natural progesterone in vaginal suppository form during the luteal phase of the menstrual cycle. Then, if conception occurs, progesterone suppositories are prescribed daily for the first 12 weeks of pregnancy. The average dosage is 50 milligrams of progesterone twice a day, but some women will be given a stronger prescription of 100 milligrams of progesterone taken 2 or even 3 times a day. Some doctors will also prescribe clomiphene citrate prior to conception, which will increase the amount of progesterone throughout the early stages of pregnancy. The progesterone suppositories are given once the pregnancy is established. Clomiphene citrate is also associated with lower incidences of miscarriage. Progesterone supplements are successful about 80% of the time in averting another miscarriage.

Repeated miscarriages can be caused by a scrambled LH (luteinizing hormone) surge. Normally, the LH surge occurs just prior to ovulation, but in some women, the surge can take place at the beginning of the cycle (common in women suffering from polycystic ovarian syndrome (PCO). The treatment is to be placed on a urofollitropin (pure FSH) or a GnRH analogue. This is still in the experimental stages, but studies show that this treatment is promising.

Between 20% and 25% of all repeated miscarriages are due to immunological problems. The woman's immune system causes her body to reject the fetus as foreign tissue for the same reason transplant patients reject organs. In this case, the mother's body is rejecting the father's antigens (a.k.a. paternal antigens) that make up the developing fetus. This problem can often be solved through either passive immunization (injecting the mother with the father's antibodies prior to conception) or active immunization (injecting white blood cells from both the mother and father into the mother's body before conception). In either case, the point of this treatment is for the mother's body to get used to his cells so that they recognize the fetus later on as friendly. Some clinics report about a 70% success rate using this method. Usually, giving the mother only paternal white blood cells yields the best results.

Other immunological causes involve women who produce antibodies that indirectly cause clotting in blood vessels that lead to the developing fetus. The fetus is deprived of nutrients and dies in utero, which triggers a miscarriage. There are no definitive treatments for this, although some clinics are looking into combining asprin, corticosteroids, or anticoagulants such as *heparin*.

About 15% of all repeated miscarriages are caused by a uterine structural problem, where tissue interferes with fetal development. This is usually correctable with surgery, depending on the severity of the defect. About 3% of repeated miscarriages are caused by an "incompetent cervix." This problem leads to second trimester miscarriages and can be prevented by stitching up the cervix. While about 5% of repeated miscarriages (as opposed to single episodes) are caused by chromosomal abnormalities, this is not a "correctable" problem, but a "luck of the draw" cause. It is also the cause of most first-time miscarriages, which occur once in six normal pregnancies. In this case, couples need to keep trying until they strike a good mix of chromosomes.

Ectopic Pregnancy (a.k.a. Tubal Pregnancy)

An ectopic pregnancy occurs when the fetus fails to implant itself in the uterus and starts to develop in the fallopian tube. Sometimes the embryo can even develop on the ovary or in the abdomen, and in this case, it's known as an *abdominal pregnancy*, which *has* been known to go to term (but it's extremely rare). If an ectopic pregnancy goes undetected, it strains the tube, which isn't designed to expand like the uterus. Then, anywhere between six to eight weeks after conception, the embryo will cause severe abdominal pain and possible vaginal bleeding. If the pain is more pronounced on one side, this is a textbook symptom of ectopic pregnancy.

Ectopic pregnancies are very dangerous. If your tube ruptures, you could suffer severe internal bleeding, which is a life-threatening situation. If you suffer sharp abdominal cramps or pains on one side, the pain may start out as a dull ache that gets more severe with time. Neck pains and shoulder pains are also common. You may also have a menstrual type of bleeding along with the pain, but the pain is the most *obvious* sign.

The problem with ectopic pregnancies is that often women don't realize they're pregnant until they have one. So, if you're trying to get pregnant or are not practicing birth control and notice any kind of unexplained abdominal pain, get yourself to a doctor as soon as you can to get it checked out.

Women in high-risk groups for ectopic pregnancies generally:

- have intrauterine devices (IUDs);
- have a history of PID;
- have a history of pelvic surgery (scarring may block the tube and prevent the egg from leaving);
- have a history of ectopic pregnancy;
- were pregnant as a result of assisted conception techniques, where gametes or embryos have been injected into their fallopian tubes; or
- have endometriosis (also see chapter 2).

If you have symptoms of ectopic pregnancy, follow the instructions outlined in the "Emergency Procedures" section below. Your doctor will check the *human chorionic gonadotropin (HCG)* hormone levels in your blood to see if they're elevated (a pregnancy test). An ultrasound will be done to check the condition of the uterus and fallopian tubes. Once an ectopic pregnancy is confirmed, *you will need emergency surgery by a skilled surgeon.* The surgery involves removing the embryo from your fallopian tube. This is delicate surgery, and you'll want someone who is capable of saving your fallopian tube *if possible.* Sometimes this isn't possible, and your fallopian tube will need to be removed (known as a *salpingectomy*). Depending on the progression of the pregnancy, you may need one ovary removed as well (known as an *oophorectomy*). You'll then need to recuperate for at least a week from surgery. After surgery, you'll need to have another blood test to make sure no embryonic tissue is left. Usually, women go on to have normal pregnancies afterward. You'll need to have at least two periods before you try again. If you have only one fallopian tube, or one ovary, it will "pick up the slack" and you'll ovulate regularly.

Although the incidence of ectopic pregnancy has increased, the fatalities from it have *decreased*. This is largely due to earlier diagnosis. Many surgeons can safely remove the embryo, preserving the tube, through *laparoscopy* (operating with a thin telescopic instrument with the aid of a video camera) instead of doing abdominal surgery, which is more invasive. There are currently studies looking into treating ectopic pregnancy with drugs, a hopeful treatment for the future. In addition, some ectopic pregnancies can be diagnosed *before* there are any symptoms, simply by checking blood levels of progesterone and beta subunits of hCG. Transvaginal ultrasound and uterine curettage are also helpful diagnostic tools.

Today, ectopic pregnancies, once a fairly rare occurrence, are considered fairly common. Between 1970 and 1987, the incidence of ectopic pregnancies rose from 18,000 to *88,000,* a *huge* increase. They now account for 1.5% of all pregnancies in the United States alone.

The consequences of an ectopic pregnancy may be upsetting. Over half of the women who aren't fortunate enough to have the ectopic diagnosed early will not conceive again, and between 10 and 15% of all ectopic sufferers will have a repeat episode.

What researchers *do* know is that lifestyle seems to play a large role in ectopic pregnancy risk. Women who smoke *less* than 10 cigarettes a day have been found in some studies to have a 40% greater risk of ectopic pregnancy. Women who smoke more than 30 cigarettes a day are five times more likely to have an ectopic pregnancy. Nicotine affects the mobility of the fallopian tubes. This may delay implantation because the tube contractions (which move the embryo along into the uterus) are affected by estrogen levels, which smoking seems to reduce. In addition, smokers can't fight off infections as well as nonsmokers, which puts them more at risk to certain STDs, which can lead to PID. Again, the increase in chlamydia and PID *directly* corresponds to the rise in ectopic pregnancies. One recent British study revealed that 76% of women who had ectopic pregnancies also had antibodies for chlamydia.

Emergency Procedures

What's the definition of an emergency at this stage? Heavy bleeding; severe pain (cramps or abdominal); sudden, severe vomiting that doesn't seem to be related to your morning sickness; and a loss of consciousness. If you're taken by surprise by the symptoms and feel they are severe, immediately call either your regular gynecologist's or primary care physician's office. If it's during business hours, ask the receptionist or answering service what hospital he or she practices at (each will be affiliated with a hospital). Inform the doctor that you will *meet* him or her there and that you're leaving now! *Then, get yourself to an emergency unit of that hospital ASAP.* If you can't drive yourself or find someone to take you, by all means call 911 and *request an ambulance.* If it's after hours, there should be a recorded message at your doctor's office that gives out an emergency number and the address of the hospital he or she is affiliated with. If you're well enough to go to emergency on your own, have someone (friend, mother, spouse, neighbor) call that emergency number and arrange for the doctor to meet you at the hospital. If you're going by ambulance, the ambulance staff will call for you. If for some reason you can't get hold of any doctor, and he or she does not have prerecorded emergency instructions, get yourself to the emergency unit of *any* hospital ASAP either on your own or by ambulance. Once you're there and being looked after, the hospital will sort everything out and find the doctor and appropriate hospital for you. Never *wait* for the doctor to call you back. Just get moving!

As you may have noticed, the first trimester carries a number of important issues you need to be aware of. By the second trimester, however, the risk of pregnancy loss drops dramatically, while many of the first-trimester symptoms vanish. (Unfortunately, some of the symptoms listed earlier in the chapter make their first appearance in the second trimester!) But as the pregnancy progresses, other issues tend to surface, such as sexual concerns, placental problems, preterm labor, and so on. Let's move on . . .

4

T2 Health
(Trimester 2)

Once your pregnancy has progressed to the fourth month, the risk of complications decreases considerably; miscarriages at this stage, known as late miscarriage, account for less than 25% of *all* miscarriages. Moreover, ectopic pregnancies are rarely discovered beyond the 12th week. It is at this stage that you'll begin to look pregnant, rather than just be mistaken for "chubby." Most women will begin to feel a little less nauseated at this point, too, but morning sickness occasionally persists well into the second trimester or even throughout the third trimester. You may also have developed some of the conditions discussed in chapter 2. Again, these diseases range from diabetes to thyroid problems. All of these diseases are dependent on family histories, and a range of other factors. You'll begin having "official" prenatal exams, which will include testing of your blood sugar levels because of the frequency of gestational diabetes's developing at this stage. You'll also begin to go for various prenatal tests, depending on your age and risk group. (Prenatal testing is covered separately in chapter 5.)

How Does It Feel?

When there *is* an end to morning sickness, you'll begin to feel better in some ways but decidedly more "pregnant" in others. By now, your waist will have expanded considerably and you won't be able to fit into many of your prepregnancy clothes. You'll begin to feel fetal movement, sometimes called quickening, in the early part of the second trimester (around week 20). This date is important to note because it will help your doctor date the pregnancy more accurately.

At this point, your entire circulatory system is changing. Your total blood volume increases, your bone marrow produces more blood corpuscles, and your heart will be changing position and increasingly slightly in size. You may notice that you're salivating more frequently, which is sometimes associated with nausea or is more pronounced if you're nauseous. You may sweat more as well.

Most women tend to feel very healthy during this trimester, in part because they actually feel the pregnancy and therefore tend to relax. They feel as though everything is "normal" and as it should be. The fetus will grow tremendously during this stage and increase in length from 3 inches to 14! By the 27th week, the fetus will weigh a little more than 2 pounds.

At this stage, the weight of your uterus increases 20 times, *while the bulk of your weight gain will take place after the 20th week.* (See section on weight in chapter 3.) As your abdominal area stretches, you may notice stretch marks, lines with pinkish or reddish streaks that appear across your stomach. Your skin may also be drier. There are other symptoms that might creep up, such as iron-deficient anemia and a host of other problems that vary from woman to woman. Here's the alphabetical breakdown of symptoms and changes that take place during the second trimester.

The ABCs

Abdominal itchiness

You may feel an itching around your abdominal wall. This is a very common complaint in pregnancy that can start at this stage, but tends to occur more frequently in the third trimester. The most pronounced itching, burning, and sometimes even numbness or pain tends to localize around the upper ribs and breastbone. This is a far more severe symptom in multiple-birth pregnancies.

Appetite

By about 17 weeks, the nausea will probably have gone away, and you may begin to experience food cravings and an increased appetite. At the same time, you may also be plagued by heartburn, indigestion, and constipation. See the section on heartburn on page 107 and the section on constipation in chapter 3.

Bowels

Constipation often gets worse as the pregnancy progresses. A high-fiber diet (discussed with your doctor and/or nutritionist) will help this. Even so, hemorrhoids may become unavoidable at this point because of pressure on your pelvic organs, and the dilation of veins in your rectum. Try propping your feet up on a stool when you move your bowels. For remedies, Preparation H , petroleum jelly, or vitamin E oil all work fine. Also see the "Constipation" and "Hemorrhoids" sections in chapter 3.

Braxton Hicks contractions

These are uterine contractions most common in the third trimester, but they can also occur sometime during the second trimester. These contractions are not signs of labor, and are mild and irregular; they're sometimes called practice labor. Each contraction lasts between 20 and 30 seconds, and they usually stop after one or two hours. During true labor, the cervix dilates and the labor contractions intensify as time goes on, something that doesn't happen with Braxton Hicks contractions.

Breasts

By the midpoint in your pregnancy, your breasts will have become fully functional and ready for breastfeeding. Around the 19th to 20th week, your nipples will secrete a yellowish liquid known as *colostrum,* a type of "pre-milk."

Carpal tunnel syndrome

Carpal tunnel syndrome refers to a type of "wrist syndrome" in which nerves in the wrist become compressed. Conditions that cause water retention (or edema), such as pregnancy, can contribute to nerve compression. When the nerves in the wrist are compressed, all feeling in your hand can be blocked. Symptoms of carpal tunnel syndrome are numbness, tingling, or burning pain in the middle and index fingers and thumb. In more severe cases, all of your fingers may be affected, and numbness can sometimes extend to the elbow.

During pregnancy, the problem is treated by wearing a splint; after delivery, the problem will often just correct itself as fluid levels in the body drop. If the problem persists after delivery, minor surgery can correct the problem and restore all feeling to your hand. If you're pregnant and perform occupational tasks that place you more at risk for carpal tunnel syndrome, there's a greater chance that you'll experience this problem. Just stay alert to the symptoms and report them to your doctor.

Continued discomforts

All the following discomforts, discussed separately in chapter 3, may either persist, or only first appear at this point. Common discomforts include: backaches, constipation, shortness of breath (dyspnea), numbness in your legs or arms caused by shifting posture, pain around your pubic area, sore ribs, leg cramps, gas, and flatulence. The reasons for these discomforts have to do with your expanding uterus, which puts pressure on your lower back area and legs and pushes up your stomach. This interferes with indigestion and rubs your ribs and upper chest the "wrong way."

Edema (water retention)

Classic edema symptoms are swollen feet, ankles and, fingers. This happens because the growing uterus puts pressure on your lower extremities, which forces water into the tissue around your feet and ankles.

Increased amounts of progesterone in your body also cause you to retain more water, which is why many women become bloated just before their periods. There's not too much you can do about water retention other than avoiding salty foods. If you're tempted to take a diuretic, *don't*. See "Urinary Frequency" in chapter 3.

Depending upon the severity of the edema, you could become prone to toxemia (preeclampsia or eclampsia, discussed in chapter 2).

"Happy hormones"

By weeks 13 and 14, your energy level will shift from fatigue to peppiness. You're not only putting on more weight, which gives you caloric energy, but much of the nausea and vomiting that has exhausted you so far, begins to taper off by this point. Your hormone levels are also extremely high, contributing to this excess energy. Sometimes the second trimester is dubbed "happy hormone time" because of this. Finally, you will begin to feel the baby move at this stage, which will make you excited about the pregnancy in a new way. Everything's "working," and your pregnancy is feeling normal and even miraculous to you.

Heartburn

Women can experience heartburn all throughout pregnancy. It most commonly occurs in the first trimester (discussed briefly in chapter 3) or begins at some point in the second trimester and continues until the end of the pregnancy.

Heartburn is a burning sensation in the middle of your chest or upper digestive tract. It's caused by progesterone, which relaxes the muscle that controls the opening at the top of the stomach. Progesterone also causes the stomach, which is pressed upwards by the growing fetus, to empty more slowly. The bottom line is that the stomach doesn't work as well as it should. Here are some tips that might help:

- Avoid fatty and greasy foods, carbonated drinks, processed meats, and junk food. Ask your nutritionist to recommend a heartburn-friendly diet for you.
- Eat slowly and chew your food very well before you swallow.

This will give the enzymes in your saliva a chance to work better and help to break down the food, which will relieve some of the digestive workload from your stomach.

- Try not to eat later in the evening (after 8 p.m.) when you're less active.

Low blood pressure

Although some women worry about high blood pressure at this stage, the opposite can also occur. Low blood pressure is not to be confused with low blood sugar (hypoglycemia), discussed in chapter 3, but it can cause similar symptoms, such as dizziness and feelings of faintness. Fainting is more likely to occur if you've been standing for long periods of time. As for "treatment," there isn't anything you can do other than shifting your positions: lie down, if possible, or sit with your head down between your knees and avoid standing in one place for prolonged periods.

Nosebleeds

By this point, *your blood volume has increased by about 40%,* which will put pressure on the veins in your nose and may cause them to bleed. (See chapter 3 for more details.) Keep a little petroleum jelly in each nostril to help prevent dryness, which can trigger a nosebleed.

Skin changes

Many women will notice changes in their skin at this point in the pregnancy. Dark blotches may occur on the face as a result of increased levels of estrogen and progesterone, which stimulate the production of melanin, a skin pigment. Sometimes women also develop a darkened area on their face in the form of a butterfly pattern, called *chloasma.*

Elsewhere, you may notice the areola on your breasts darkening, and you may get a dark line running from your navel to your pubic hair. This line is called the *linea negra,* which will usually go away; darkened aureola are permanent, however.

The consistency of your skin and hair may also change and become either very dry or very oily.

Finally, if you have any moles on your body, they may become darker and larger. This usually isn't anything to worry about, but because of the increased incidence of melanoma and other skin cancers, this must not go unchecked by your doctor. If a mole changes in size or color, get it looked at; you may want to consider removing the mole altogether, which is a simple procedure that can be performed in your doctor's office.

Vaginal discharge

As discussed in chapter 3, a thin, milky, odorless discharge known as *leukorrhea* will have developed and begins to get heavier around now. You may need to wear lightday pads for this. Yeast infections may also begin to plague you and can persist throughout your pregnancy.

Veins

You'll notice numerous changes in your veins at this stage, due to the increase in your blood volume. See the separate section on venous changes below.

Weight

You will have gained a significant amount of weight during the second trimester. The average weight gain by this point totals between 10 to 15 pounds. You waist and hips will thicken, so now is the time to change into those maternity clothes! See the section in chapter 3 on nutrition, fitness, and weight for more details.

Yeast infections, urinary frequency, and UTIs

These are discussed in detail in chapter 3. Urinary frequency will increase as your uterus enlarges and puts pressure on your bladder. Yeast infections and urinary tract infections are common problems in pregnancy that can be treated with antifungal medications (for yeast) or antibiotics (for urinary tract infections) safe to use during pregnancy.

The Venous Chronicles

Since your blood volume has now increased by *40-45%*, your veins may change drastically, but this is a normal part of pregnancy. Venous changes range from unsettling blue lines under the skin around the breasts or abdomen to bona fide varicose veins. The blue lines you're seeing are just more prominent and expanded veins. They've expanded because your blood supply has increased, which is necessary to nourish the fetus.

Some women get spidery, purplish lines up and down their thighs, known as "superficial varicosities." "Spider nevi" or *telangiectases* may also develop, which are similar lines on the chest. Both result from hormonal changes. These lines might fade or disappear after pregnancy. If they don't, they can be remedied through minor cosmetic procedures.

As for varicose veins, these tend to run in families. The veins carry blood back from all your extremities to your heart. They are designed with valves to prevent the blood from flowing backward in the veins. The valves need to work against gravity when they're carrying blood up the leg. Sometimes the vein valves are faulty or missing, which causes the blood to collect in areas where the gravity is most pronounced: the legs, rectum, or even vulva. These blood *pools* in the legs are noticeable, clumpy, and painful. Unfortunately, an expanded blood volume and an increase in progesterone just makes the condition more pronounced or will initially trigger it in women who haven't yet suffered from varicose veins but who are vulnerable to them.

Sometimes the only sign of varicose veins is the appearance of faint bluish lines in the areas where the blood pools. A bulging can crop up anywhere from the ankles to the vulva. In more severe cases, *thrombophlebitis* can develop, which means "inflammation of the vein due to blood clot." When a clot develops in a vein, this is known as *venous thrombosis*.

Clotting usually occurs in the postpartum period, but varicose veins can develop at any point in the pregnancy. The treatment revolves around prevention: maintaining a healthy pregnancy weight (overeating can worsen varicose veins); raising your legs while lying down (stick a pillow under them to get the blood flow moving); wearing support pantyhose (this keeps the blood circulating); avoiding restrictive clothing such as tight belts, snug shoes, garters, girdles, and so on; and daily walks (about 20–30 minutes a day).

Hemorrhoids, discussed in chapter 3, may also develop. Hemorrhoids are basically *prolapsed veins* inside your rectum. Here's how they form: You have three primary veins around your rectum and when you become constipated (as you will be during pregnancy), your feces become hard, which causes you to push harder when you need to defecate. The continuous pushing causes the veins in your rectum to prolapse (fall down) and protrude outside of your rectum. As the pregnancy progresses, the pressure that the baby's head places on your rectal area only increases, which aggravates the hemorrhoids. Hemorrhoids are generally harmless, but alarming. There are two kinds of hemorrhoids that may develop: a black hemorrhoid, caused by an old blood clot (your hemorrhoid once bled, clotted, and has now turned black from old, stale blood), and a bright red hemorrhoid, caused by a continuous circulation of blood through it (new blood keeps passing through the hemorrhoid, not giving it a chance to clot). The best thing you can do is carry around a tube of topical anesthetic, lubricate your fingers with it, and physically tuck these rectal veins back in the rectum whenever you defecate. See chapter 3 for more information on hemorrhoids.

Twice the Size, Double the Discomfort

As with the first trimester, multiple fetuses usually *double* your discomfort. However, there are some women who feel wonderful during this phase and seem to blossom and glow about their double "treasures." *But don't count on it!*

The most common physical symptoms for "multiple" moms are insomnia, exhaustion, a more severe version of the normal second-trimester symptoms (including more severe vein changes), aches and pains (back, lower legs), water retention (swollen hands, feet, ankles), prolonged nausea, and the inability to walk more than a short distance (although this tends to be more of a problem for most multiple-birth pregnancies in the third trimester).

Much of the extra discomfort is due to an enormous increase in your blood volume, necessary to service two placentas. In addition, you'll be putting on considerably more weight than mothers carrying single fetuses. The normal range of weight gain for multiple births is anywhere from less than 30 pounds to more than 80 pounds. *However, it's important to keep in mind that when you're carrying more than one child, it's better to err on the side of overweight than underweight!* This will ensure that both (or all) fetuses are getting the best possible nourishment.

Of course, some of you reading this section may be carrying more than one fetus *but not realize it yet*. This brings us to the question every pregnant woman asks at this stage: *"Is it twins?"* The answer to this is determined during your first prenatal exam (or first exam in the second trimester, if you've been seeing your doctor throughout the first trimester).

The Prenatal Exam

As discussed in chapter 1, you'll initially need to be screened for sexually transmitted diseases (STDs), genetic disorders, and other diseases, as well as have a complete physical and pelvic exam. This can be done either just before you plan to get pregnant or once you first discover the pregnancy. Once all of these things are in order, you technically don't need to have a prenatal exam until at least 12 weeks into the pregnancy. Depending on your healthcare system or plan, many obstetricians won't even schedule an appointment until this point. However, if you're seeing a private physician, he or she may encourage you to have a prenatal exam in the first trimester. This is always a good idea because the sooner you see the doctor, the more accurately your pregnancy can be dated.

Whether you have your first prenatal exam at three months or four months, you'll begin to see the doctor every month thereafter and sometimes more often if your pregnancy is a difficult one. By the end of the third trimester, you'll be seeing your doctor every week.

The prenatal exam usually lasts about 10–15 minutes and consists of the following:

- Weight and blood pressure check (via scale and blood pressure instrument). This is a good time to bring up dietary questions and request an appointment with a nutritionist, if you haven't already.
- Urinalysis for sugar and protein levels (via urine sample) to detect either gestational diabetes or protein in your urine, a possible sign of toxemia.
- Fetal heartbeat check (by putting a stethoscope to the outside of your uterus.) See the "Heartbeat" section below.
- Measuring the size of your uterus. (Your doctor can do this just by feeling the outside of your uterus. Based on the size of your uterus, he or she will also correct or confirm the original due date you calculated). The date of your last period is used to determine whether the fetus is growing at a consistent rate. Generally, the size of your uterus is equal to the age of the fetus. So if you seem larger or smaller than you should be, you may need an ultrasound test done to determine the true length of the pregnancy or whether you're carrying more than one fetus.
- Checking the height of the *top* of your uterus (also called the fundus).
- A visual inspection for edema and vein changes.
- Questions about your symptoms.
- Suggested remedies or safe medications for your symptoms, and possible follow-up visits in between your monthly checkups.
- Possible blood tests for certain conditions depending on your age, weight and symptoms. (This may also include checking hormone levels, which is discussed separately on page 115.)

You shouldn't need an internal exam during a routine prenatal exam unless your doctor suspects a problem and needs to check your cervix for some reason (such as a history of an incompetent cervix, for example, discussed on page 53). In an unremarkable pregnancy, this exam will not change very much from month to month.

King-Size or Twins?

Since we know more today about good nutrition and the causes of low birthweight (such as smoking and drinking), many women are giving birth to 8-, 9-, and even 10- pound babies. However, you may naturally wonder whether your size indicates one king-size baby, or twins. There are several ways your practitioner can detect twins at this stage.

Checking your alpha fetoprotein (AFP) levels

See chapter 5 about this for more details. Elevated AFP is a sign of twins and will need to be followed up with an ultrasound.

The heartbeat

By the beginning of this trimester, your doctor will be able to detect the fetal heartbeat with two special stethoscope-like devices. In the past, a fetal stethoscope, called a *fetoscope* (which can detect the heartbeat until 20 weeks), was all that was used to check the heartbeat, but now a more advanced instrument called a *Doptone,* which uses ultrasound, is far more sensitive. The problem with detecting twin heartbeats, however, is that sometimes one twin's position can muffle the heartbeat of its roommate.

If two heartbeats *are* suspected, at about the 18th week, two examiners (your doctor and a midwife or a midwife and nurse) will listen to the fetal heartbeat(s) *simultaneously* and count the beats separately using either two Doptones or one Doptone and one fetoscope. Often, two heartbeats will beat to a different pattern. Your pulse should be taken as well, so your examiners don't confuse your heartbeat with the heartbeat of a fetus.

Ultrasound

Discussed more fully in chapter 5, ultrasound will always confirm multiple fetuses, if they are suspected.

If you've just discovered that you're carrying more than one fetus, you'll graduate to a high-risk pregnancy and will probably see your doctor every two weeks instead of the usual monthly visit. (Please review chapter 2 for more details.) If you're working, you'll need to go on maternity leave at around the fifth month. Studies in Scandinavian countries show that women carrying twins (or more) increase their chances of premature labor if they continue working beyond the fifth month. Women carrying twins who *stopped* working after five months had a much lower incidence of premature labor. In North America, the "Scandinavian rules" are now used by all obstetricians caring for multiple-birth patients.

The Second-Trimester Lab Package

While some of you will not have to have any blood tests done, many of you will. Typical things checked for in blood tests at this point are your white-blood-cell and red-blood-cell count, hemoglobin, blood type, and Rh factor. Some doctors may also choose to screen for rubella, chlamydia, syphilis, HIV, hepatitis B, and possibly toxoplasmosis. Screenings of this type, however, will be done only if you neglected to do so before or if your doctor suspects exposure to some of these infections. (All of these are discussed in detail in chapter 2)

In addition, many of you will have an *alpha fetoprotein* (AFP) test or a "triple screen," consisting of a blood test that checks your AFP levels, hCG levels and levels of a serum estrogen called estriol. This test screens for neural tube defects in the fetus such as *spina bifida* (an open spinal cord); multiple fetuses; and hCG levels. It also monitors fetal activity. This test is discussed separately in chapter 5.

Sex and the Pregnant Woman

As your pregnancy progresses, you'll naturally have some questions about sex during pregnancy. What's safe? Is there anything you *shouldn't* be doing? What's *normal*? How will the pregnancy affect your partner's sexual desire for you? This section, which is also included in chapter 6, is designed to answer all of your concerns and may shed some light on issues you may *not* have thought about.

In the Beginning

There's nothing sexual that you can't do during the first trimester. The only women who may need to be cautious about their sexual activities at this point are women with a history of repeated miscarriages (three or more). During orgasm, uterine contractions may lift off a newly implanted embryo, but this is only a very small risk. However, thrusting will not bother the pregnancy at all. You can have vigorous and enthusiastic sex as often as you like at this stage. If you *do* notice spotting after sex, consult your doctor about it.

Let There Be Light

Certain sexual positions may become uncomfortable for you, while others may become very arousing; this is perfectly natural. Many women might suddenly be uncomfortable with the missionary position because they'll feel anxious about the weight the male is putting on their abdominal areas. Technically, this weight will not in any way harm the fetus, but if you're anxious about it, you won't enjoy yourself.

If this is your first child, don't be surprised by odd reactions to sex from your partner. He may feel as if the baby "can see him" having sex with you. He may also feel that he is hurting you in some way, and may wish to abstain from sex. The solution? Take your partner to your doctor's office with you, and have your doctor explain how the baby's protected. Or, start a conversation with "My doctor told me that sex..."

On the upside, your breasts will become fuller, firmer, and your nipples will enlarge. Because of this, you'll not only feel sexier but will look sexier to your partner, who will most likely say "let there be light" the next time you try to switch off the night-table lamp. Being on top may be the best position for you, and your partner can play with your newly-enlarged breasts, as enlarged nipples become even larger as they become erect with arousal. Have fun and enjoy it while it lasts. (This is a particular treat for normally small-breasted women.) Since nipple stimulation releases the hormone *oxytocin* into your bloodstream, which causes uterine muscles to contract, some women may be concerned that nipple stimulation later in the pregnancy (from the fifth month on) may lead to premature labor. Relax. To date, studies regarding the danger of nipple stimulation during pregnancy have been inconclusive. A frank discussion about your concerns with your doctor or midwife might be a good idea if you're concerned or have a history of preterm labor. (Breasts are discussed in detail in chapter 9.)

As a general rule at all times, and particularly during pregnancy, *do* get into the habit of emptying your bladder after sex. This helps wash out harmful bacteria that may have entered you with your partner's penis, which in turn can cause urinary tract infections (UTIs).

As You Get Larger (13–24 weeks)

Many women begin to feel very sexual and feminine with their pregnant bodies. Because of this, your libido may actually increase at this stage. This is normal and healthy, so enjoy yourself. At the same time, you may also have hemorrhoids and other not-so-fun symptoms, and will obviously be larger. Again, being on top during sex is a good position at this point; it provides for better breast play, allows better control of the thrusting, and relieves pressure from your rectal area, which may be sensitive. Another good position at this stage is rear entry. While not glamorous, this position allows your abdomen to rest comfortably on the bed, leaving your hands free to stimulate your partner and his hands free to stimulate *you*. Also, since your breasts will be more sensitive at this stage, rear entry allows them to rest comfortably on the bed, instead of being pressed against or pulled on.

A common problem with being pregnant and sexually aroused is partner incompatibility. He may become more weary of sex as you get larger, feeling somehow "sacrilegious" about having intercourse. Or the feeling of hurting you or the baby may resurface or persist as the pregnancy progresses. There *is* a real solution to your dilemma in this case: masturbation. Mutual, solo, any time of the day or night, masturbation does wonders for a pregnant woman's sex life. It's common, normal, and very healthy. It takes the pressure off your partner and allows you to focus on pleasuring yourself.

Is there any time during the second trimester when you shouldn't have sex? Yes. If you're bleeding for any reason, have bloody discharge, or are feeling labor contractions (not to be confused with the Braxton Hicks contractions discussed above), don't have sex.

The only other consequence of sex during the second trimester is that if, for some reason, you have a missed abortion (the fetus dies in utero, but does not expel itself), sex may trigger the uterus to contract and expel the fetus. However, sex does not *cause* the missed abortion; it only helps to expel it. This distinction is important because some women may be inclined to believe that their sexual activity has somehow caused the death of the fetus, which is *not* the case.

Anal Knowledge

As you may already know, anal sex today is what oral sex was 20 years ago: It's very common. As you may also know, anal sex provides a thriving organic garden for STDs of every kind to grow in. Why? During anal sex, small tears in the sensitive rectal area can bleed. This blood-to-semen contact can be a real killer, and is why HIV is so easily transmitted through anal sex. What makes anal sex *more* dangerous during pregnancy is largely ignorance and myth.

Myth: I heard you can only get STDs with vaginal intercourse. To protect the baby, I'll have anal intercourse instead.

Fact: Wrong! Wrong! Wrong! There is such a thing as anal herpes and anal gonorrhea, both terrible fates for any pregnant woman. Genital warts, caused by the *human papillomavirus (HPV)*, can also form around your rectum, aggravating your condition as well.

Myth: "C'mon, honey, let's do it this way. It will be safer for the baby. You'll see, you'll like it once we get into it . . . ."

Fact: As soon as your partner hears you say no, wait, stop, or ouch, make sure he's *out* of there! Once you feel discomfort, your rectum will tighten, which means there's a greater chance of doing serious damage to your rectal tissues. This will aggravate any discomforts in your pregnancy even more. In a worst case scenario, tears become so bad that tearing of your bowel can occur. The result: Feces may bypass your rectum altogether and come out through your vagina, which can bring on vaginal infections of nightmarish proportion!

Anal sex rules during pregnancy

The best choice is to abstain at all times. However, if you do choose to have anal sex in a stable, monogamous relationship, use caution, consideration, and a lot of lubricant. Otherwise, make sure your partner uses two condoms (i.e., "doublebag" it) and a lot of lubricant.

Things that Can Go Wrong

When something goes wrong in the pregnancy at this point, it usually has to do with either *your* health, be it an infection, structural problem, or injury, or a problem with the placenta, both of which might trigger a miscarriage or premature labor,

Bleeding

This time, light or spotty bleeding is often caused by an increasingly sensitive cervix, which may be irritated in an internal exam (if you've had one for any reason) or during sexual intercourse. At any rate, you'll need to notify your doctor immediately about the bleeding. Heavier bleeding at this stage can also be caused by either a low-lying placenta (*placenta previa*) or the premature separation of the placenta (*abruptio placenta*), but these problems are more common in the third trimester and are discussed in more detail in chapter 6. Bleeding can also be a sign that you're losing the pregnancy or that you're experiencing premature labor, discussed on page 121.

Late Miscarriage

Between the third month and 20th week of pregnancy, a spontaneous abortion is known as a late miscarriage. The symptoms are similar to those of a first-trimester miscarriage. In many cases, the condition known as an incompetent, or weak, cervix is responsible. This is when the cervix dilates prematurely and cannot hold in the fetus. For the most part, the causes of an incompetent cervix are unknown, but trauma to the cervix as a result of infection, for example, can trigger premature dilation. An incompetent cervix is also more common if you're a DES daughter, due to a possible malformation of the cervix. (See chapter 2 for more information on DES daughters.)

If an incompetent cervix is caught early enough, as may be the case if you've had repeated miscarriages, the cervix can be stitched up, after which, at around 38 weeks or prior to labor, the stitches can be removed and a normal vaginal birth can take place. Some stitching techniques are permanent, however, causing a cesarean section to be necessary.

If the miscarriage is inevitable and can't be prevented, a D & C can be performed up until the 20th week. A miscarriage after 20 weeks is no longer a miscarriage and becomes either a premature birth or a stillbirth, discussed in chapter 6. Under these circumstances, you'll need to follow the steps outlined under "Emergency Procedures" in chapter 3.

Premature Labor

Premature labor is characterized by contractions accompanied by vaginal bleeding or discharge or even a vaginal pressure, anywhere from the 20th week to the 37th week. Premature rupture of the membranes (the amniotic sac) occurs in 20–30% of all premature deliveries and is a sign that something is wrong as well. Other symptoms of premature labor are menstrual-like cramps, with possible diarrhea, nausea, or indigestion, lower back pain, and all the other symptoms of labor discussed in chapter 7.

Between 5 and 8% of all deliveries are premature. The health of the premature newborn greatly depends on exactly *how* premature the delivery is, what kind of neonatal care is available, the weight of the newborn, and how developed he or she is. Babies born before 25 weeks (weighing slightly more than 2 pounds) have about a 50% chance of surviving, *assuming* that they're receiving appropriate treatment in a neonatal unit. However, this statistic also takes into account children who survive with severe disabilities, such as cerebral palsy, and forms of mental retardation. When the newborn weighs 3 pounds or more, his/her survival rate jumps to about 95%.

What causes premature labor at this stage?

For the most part, the causes of premature labor at this stage are unknown, but the factors that are known to trigger it include:

- *Poor general health.* Cigarette smoking and inadequate nutrition can increase your risk of premature labor.
- *Diabetes and/or thyroid problems.* If these conditions have *not* been treated appropriately, your risk of premature labor can increase.
- *Cocaine use.* This has been cited as a definite cause of premature labor.
- *Bacterial vaginosis.* (See chapter 1)
- *Syphilis.* Syphilis can definitely trigger premature labor. (Review chapters 1 and 2 on STD screening.)
- *A garden variety of bacterial infections too numerous to list.*
- *Placental problems.* These can trigger premature labor in this trimester and are discussed in chapter 6.
- *Pylenephritis.* (See chapter 3)
- *Physical trauma, such as a bad fall.* Women in physically abusive

relationships are particularly vulnerable to premature labor at this stage. (Auto accidents are still the number-one cause of physical trauma–related miscarriages.)

What should you do?

This is an *emergency situation* and can be treated with medications that postpone the labor. As soon as you begin feeling contractions, contact your doctor immediately, then you'll need to go directly to your birthing facility or an emergency room at the nearest hospital. Follow the emergency procedures outlined in chapter 3. If your contractions are successfully halted with medication, you may be put on strict bed rest for the duration of the pregnancy.

Depending on how severe the situation is, your doctor may decide to proceed with delivery. If your membranes have ruptured, or you're having vaginal bleeding, there is no way you can stop the labor; you'll need to go ahead and deliver. If, however, you have ruptured your membranes, but are neither experiencing contractions nor any vaginal bleeding, the delivery may be postponed until the baby's lungs are mature. This is the situation in about 25% of the time.

In the worst-case scenario, the baby will be born prematurely and treated in a neonatal unit. Premature labor is more commonly a third-trimester problem. I've also provided a first-aid section called "Emergency Childbirth Procedures" in chapter 7. Please review this section for more details.

Flooding or Drought: Amniotic Fluid Problems

Your baby floats inside amniotic fluid, which surrounds and protects it. In an average pregnancy, you need to have about 2 quarts of amniotic fluid (2000 milliliters). If you have more, you have too much fluid, creating a condition known as *hydramnios,* or *polyhydramnios.* If you don't have enough fluid, a condition known as *oligohydramnios* can develop. Both conditions are dangerous, creating either a flood or drought environment for the fetus. As in our own environment, a balanced water supply is essential for its health.

You're more likely to overproduce amniotic fluid if you're carrying twins, have diabetes, or have an Rh incompatibility. Hydramnios can develop gradually or appear suddenly. The first symptoms will be related to an expansion of your uterus as a result of too much fluid. All your normal discomforts will become exaggerated. Your doctor may find it difficult to hear the baby's heartbeat as a result of too much fluid. Basically, your doctor will examine you and decide how severe your hydramnios is. He or she may decide to induce labor and deliver prematurely if you or your baby's health is in danger.

Signs of oligohydramnios may not be obvious unless an ultrasound is done to confirm it. This is a serious condition that can be caused by a few things. One cause is due to a malfunction or even absence of, the fetus's kidney. A major ingredient to healthy amniotic fluid is the fetal urine. Without it, you don't have enough fluid that provides the necessary cushioning for proper fetal development. Another cause of oligohydramnios is leakage of amniotic fluid, due to a premature rupture of membranes (more details in Chapter 7). When this happens, friction-related problems may occur and the fetal lungs may not mature normally. The condition may also occur in a post-mature baby (see chapter 6) if caught in the third trimester. The problem usually warrants being induced and delivering prematurely.

Common Second-Trimester Health Problems

One in four women will develop gestational diabetes, which is discussed in more detail in chapter 2. If you are prone to gestational diabetes, it usually occurs at this stage in the pregnancy. Currently, the American College of Obstetricians and Gynecologists (ACOG) suggests that all women over the age of 30 and women at higher risk for gestational diabetes (see chapter 2 for high-risk groups) should be screened for it in the second trimester. However, many doctors now believe that *all* women should be screened for gestational diabetes between weeks 24 and 28. If gestational diabetes remains undiagnosed, it can be very dangerous for the fetus because it will cause the fetus to gain more weight than it should at this point, increasing *your* risk of developing labor or other delivery complications as a result of the baby's size.

Toxemia, also discussed in chapter 2, will occur in about 5% of the second-trimester population. If it occurs, it will usually appear later than week 20. Thyroid disease is also a common problem that may develop at this point.

Molar Pregnancy: A Type of Placental Cancer

Roughly one in every 1,500–2,000 pregnancies in North America will develop into a *molar pregnancy,* also known as a *hydatidiform mole.* Molar pregnancies are more common in other parts of the world, however, and are most frequently reported among women in Asia, the South Pacific, and Mexico.

A molar pregnancy is an accident of fertilization. It results from a conception with an abnormal set of chromosomes. In the most common form, no embryo develops, and instead, the placenta grows to form a cluster of small cysts. If the patient miscarries and expels these cysts, they will look like clusters of grapes. Rarely, a condition called a partial molar pregnancy will occur. Here, there is a fetus, but it usually has 69 chromosomes instead of the usual 46, and will not be able to survive.

There are three ways this freakish fertilization occurs: One way is for two sperm to fertilize one egg, with the loss of the mother's chromosomes. The second way is for one sperm to enter the egg and then divide, delivering a double dose of chromosomes to the egg instead of its usual single dose. A third way would be for an abnormal sperm carrying two sets of chromosomes to fertilize the egg.

The cysts that characterize a molar pregnancy are benign but can develop into a type of cancer called *choriocarcinoma,* or cancer of the chorion, which secretes the vital growth hormone, human chorionic gonadotropin (hCG). It's imperative that a molar pregnancy is removed as soon as it's detected, unless the fetus is healthy. (Again, a healthy fetus in this situation is extremely rare.)

Symptoms

Symptoms of a molar pregnancy can begin in the first trimester, but it is often not diagnosed until the second trimester. The first sign is continuous staining. The molar pregnancy can even damage the placenta to the point of miscarriage, You might just experience what you think is a normal first- or second-trimester miscarriage, until you're examined via ultrasound, which will always confirm a molar pregnancy. In this case, bleeding will usually become heavy and a D & C will always be performed to prevent any molar tissue from being left behind.

In other cases, the bleeding can be light and the fetus may die but not expel itself. In this case, a suction abortion followed by a D & C *must* be performed.

Another sign of a molar pregnancy is very high levels of hCG, which only drop slightly over time after the pregnancy ends. Because of this, women who have had molar pregnancies will need to be watched closely for at least a year before they can become pregnant again, and should practice either oral contraception or barrier methods. If the hCG levels have dropped over the year, then it's safe to conceive again. If the hCG levels don't drop, it means that the danger of choriocarcinoma is still present, in which case and you'll need to consult an *oncologist,* or a cancer specialist.

Most women who have had a molar pregnancy can expect to have normal future pregnancies. Repeated molar pregnancies are uncommon, but you'll need to consult with your doctor as to when it's safe to conceive again, and then rule out a molar pregnancy in the first trimester via checking your hCG levels and having an ultrasound.

Vanishing Twin Syndrome

This condition used to be considered rarer than it is now thought to be. As many as 80% of all twin pregnancies (which occur in about 7 out of every 100 pregnancies) will experience a phenomenon known as vanishing twin syndrome. Here, the pregnancy starts out as a twin pregnancy, but only one fetus actually develops.

Symptoms of vanishing twin syndrome are similar to the symptoms of miscarriage (vaginal bleeding, cramps, decreased hormone levels), but then a healthy fetus may be discovered during the ultrasound. More often, though, there are no symptoms and the second twin is reabsorbed by the body, while remnants of its placenta and membrane may be delivered at the birth of the surviving twin. In some cases, remnants of a second placenta during delivery may be the only clue that a twin has "vanished."

This syndrome would likely not even have surfaced as a phenomenon if it weren't for ultrasound technology. With ultrasound, two fetuses may be detected as early as the first trimester, and then, in the second trimester, you may be told that one has vanished. This can be traumatic for many women, but an experience that is not well-documented or openly discussed. As ultrasound technology improves, more twin pregnancies will be diagnosed in the first trimester, and hence, more twins will "vanish" by the second, creating a more common pregnancy loss phenomenon as well as more information about it.

Testing . . . 1-2-3

The bulk of your prenatal testing is done during the second trimester and will include ultrasound, an alpha fetoprotein screening (AFP), and possibly amniocentesis. But many other tests are performed that you may not be aware of. The purposes behind all of these tests, deciding whether even to have tests done, waiting for the test results, and deciding to terminate the pregnancy in the event of a problem, are all topics discussed in the next chapter.

5

Prenatal Testing

In 1995, it is 10 times safer to have a child than it was in 1895. This enormous decrease in childbirth-related deaths is due to antibiotics, safe blood transfusion, and anesthesia. Consequently, prenatal testing has been developed to improve the outlook for a newborn. The point of prenatal testing is to detect potential problems early enough to create the best possible circumstances for the mother and the unborn child, whether it means having a cesarean section, having labor induced and delivering prematurely, or terminating the pregnancy.

This chapter will explain everything you need to know about prenatal testing. You'll discover which tests are appropriate, which conditions each test is designed to screen for, and what tests you'll need to confirm a problem. You'll also discover the procedure involved in terminating a second-trimester pregnancy. Since there is no test in the first trimester that can confirm a problem beyond a reasonable doubt, you must always follow up with amniocentesis, which can only be done in the second trimester. Deciding to have a first-trimester abortion *solely* based on prenatal test results is still not possible. Antepartum fetal testing is discussed in chapter 6.

Why All the Tests?

After you conceive, every possible problem is anticipated and screened for. Initially, as discussed in chapters 1 and 2, you'll be routinely screened via simple blood and urine tests for all kinds of diseases including anemia, blood sugar problems (hypoglycemia, gestational diabetes), STDs (HIV, herpes, gonorrhea, syphilis, genital warts, chlamydia), kidney disease, toxemia, Rh factor, genetic diseases (if you're at risk, the list of genetic diseases to be screened for is long and getting longer, and testing is offered to those of you with family histories or another affected child), sex-linked chromosomal problems (hemophilia, cystic fibrosis), rubella, and a host of other infections discussed in chapter 2. The results of all these tests form the rationale for whether or not to have the "big" tests, such as ultrasound, alphafetoprotein screening (AFP), and later in your pregnancy, amniocentesis. Cordocentesis and chorionic villus sampling (CVS) may also be recommended.

The "Industry Standard" Tests

All pregnant women can expect to be recommended for one AFP screening (discussed separately below). As for ultrasound, most of you will end up having at least one, but in a normal pregnancy, it's not necessarily recommended. This is discussed further below. Why are these tests, once designed exclusively for high-risk pregnancies, being used as routine tests? Progress. In the same way that upgraded computer software quickly becomes an industry standard, so do diagnostic tests in the healthcare industry. Since your doctor can now routinely screen for a lot more "stuff" with ultrasound and AFP, and both tests so far pose no documented health risks, these tests are now considered *necessary extras*. Basically, ultrasound and AFP are today what blood tests and urine tests were 30 years ago.

Amniocentesis is still reserved only for high-risk situations. If you're among one of the groups identified as high risk in chapter 2, you'll most likely be recommended for amniocentesis. Or, if the results of other, earlier tests are suspicious, amniocentesis may be recommended as a follow-up procedure either to rule out or confirm a problem. All women have a right to refuse amniocentesis for a variety of reasons outlined further on. Although some newer tests have been developed that screen for some of the same things as amniocentesis, the decision to terminate a pregnancy will still be based on amniocentesis results.

Ultrasound

In prenatal testing, ultrasound (also called ultrasonography) is the use of an echo sounder to produce a picture of the baby inside the uterus. High-frequency, low-energy sound waves are used to scan your abdomen, reflecting the fetus's outline on an electronic screen through a series of bright dots. Most pregnant women can expect to have at least one ultrasound anytime after the first trimester.

For the procedure, you will need to have a full bladder. This entails drinking copious amounts of water about an hour before the ultrasound, which will be done at the doctor's office (more likely in the United States) or birthing facility (more likely in Canada). A full bladder causes the uterus, which normally lies behind the pelvic bones, to be pushed outward. This makes the baby easier to find and see on the scan. Some jelly is rubbed all over your abdomen, and a probe (called a transducer) is placed on the jellied area and moved around. A computer translates the sound echoes into video pictures. This picture is called a sonogram. The operator will point out what the patterns in the video picture mean and will show you your baby on the screen. You should be able to see the baby moving and its heart beating from about the 6th week on. The procedure takes about 30 minutes, and you may be uncomfortable because of your full bladder. In early pregnancy (the first trimester), scanning may be done with a vaginal probe and an empty bladder.

Although many women assume that ultrasound is completely safe and harmless, we still don't know if ultrasound carries risks that have not yet been documented. Ultrasounds are important if you have a high-risk pregnancy or have encountered a problem. In these circumstances, the diagnostic benefits of ultrasound far outweigh any possible, not-yet-published risks. Many women will want the experience of ultrasound because they can actually see the child in the womb, and in most cases, feel reassured that everything is normal. However, if you're having a routine, low-risk pregnancy and you don't require an ultrasound other than for curiosity purposes, you may want to research the process more and rethink your decision. Ask your physician why he or she wants to perform an ultrasound and how frequently he or she will do one.

What Ultrasound Can Detect

Ultrasound provides a detailed visual picture of the pregnancy. Your doctor will be able to tell whether:

- the baby is growing normally;
- the baby's size conflicts with the date of the pregnancy (a too small or too large fetus can mean other problems and require possible follow-up tests);
- you're carrying multiple fetuses;
- the baby is in the correct position for delivery; and
- whether the baby has any defects or abnormality (this can be determined by week 18)

Here are some legitimate reasons for an ultrasound:

- To date the pregnancy when the date of the last menstrual period is in question or unknown. This is done between 15 and 18 weeks of pregnancy or earlier. Ultrasound for this purpose could be easily eliminated by more careful charting of menstrual periods. (In very early pregnancy, a vaginal scan would be better for this, however)
- Your doctor may suspect developmental problems. (Ultra-

sound may be a follow-up to a suspicious AFP test, discussed on page 135.)

- As a diagnostic tool to help pin down abnormal bleeding, pains, or other suspicious symptoms at any time during the pregnancy. (This is when an ultrasound may be done during the first trimester.)
- Your doctor may suspect a multiple birth.
- You are in a high-risk pregnancy category.
- Your doctor may suspect a structural problem with the uterus or other part that could cause problems during delivery.
- *You're* concerned about the baby's development. (If an ultrasound scan will relax you, do it.)

Depending on why the ultrasound is initially performed, you may need to have it repeated between 32 and 34 weeks.

Some legitimate questions to ask your doctor about the ultrasound:

1. Why do I need this ultrasound?
2. What kind of follow-up tests will I need if you find something suspicious?
3. What will we learn from the results of this particular ultrasound?
4. What are the consequences of not having this ultrasound?

Again, there's nothing wrong with having an ultrasound because it's "neat," but you don't need to have a prenatal test just because it's available.

When To Have Your First Ultrasound

Unless you're experiencing problems in the first trimester or early second trimester, you don't need the test until around the 18th week. That's because developmental or structural fetal abnormalities (a key problem you'll want detected) cannot be detected up prior to that time. If your doctor suspects twins, you'll need to have an ultrasound earlier.

Most doctors will limit your ultrasound scans to two, unless there are reasons to have more. The second scan will be done toward the end of the third trimester to make sure that the position of the baby is normal.

More than two ultrasounds in a routine pregnancy should be questioned, not because they are harmful, but because they're a waste of time and money (yours, your hospital's, your insurance company's, and/or government's). The money and time would be better spent on women who truly need ultrasounds in the event of a problem.

Alpha Fetoprotein (AFP) Screening

Also referred to as *maternal serum alpha fetoprotein screening (MSAFP)*, this is a voluntary blood test that can be performed anytime between the 14th and 20th weeks of pregnancy. It's preferable to screen at 14 weeks, though, because the sooner you have the better. This test is often referred to as the "triple screen" because in many clinics it involves three separate tests for AFP, hCG levels, and a serum estrogen called estriol. From this triple screen, a calculation can be performed that will identify whether you're at risk for a Down's syndrome pregnancy. It can also pick up Down's syndrome in women under 35.

Alpha fetoprotein is a compound normally manufactured in the liver of the fetus, and it is an important carrier of molecules in the fetus's bloodstream. This protein is known as a *glycoprotein* that can be measured in both amniotic fluid and the mother's blood (maternal serum). If the alpha fetoprotein levels are higher than usual, its possible that there may be certain birth defects, including neural tube defects such as *spina bifida*, where part of the spinal column is exposed through an opening, and *anencephaly*, where part of the skull is missing and the brain isn't formed properly. The levels would be high in this case because the protein is leaking out of a defective spinal cord. However, when the spinal cord is closed, and there is a defect of another kind, AFP would not pick it up.

It's important to note that high levels of AFP are often found in women carrying twins and when the fetus has died in utero. There are also many false positive results with this test. As a result, a positive AFP is always followed up with an ultrasound if you haven't done one yet. The ultrasound will tell the doctor the gestational date of the fetus and rule out or confirm twins. If the gestational date of the fetus is older than was previously believed, the AFP will need to be recalculated to account for the fetus's age. If the gestational age is correct, and there is a single fetus, then the AFP is repeated before an amniocentesis is recommended. If the second AFP is still abnormal, both an ultrasound and amniocentesis will be done to confirm or rule out a suspected problem.

All you need to do is roll up your sleeve and give some blood. The results are usually ready in 3–5 days.

High AFP Levels

For every 1,000 women who take this test, roughly 50 will be told that their AFP levels are suspiciously high. Out of those 50, only two will actually have a child with neural tube defects. As for the remaining 48:

- some will have a normal AFP level the second time around;
- some will have inaccurately dated the pregnancy (sometimes a growth scan may be done to monitor the baby's progress in this case);
- some will be carrying multiple fetuses;
- some will have babies with other forms of defects; and
- some will have perfectly normal children, never finding out why their AFP levels were elevated.

If your second AFP test is normal, an ultrasound may be done anyway just to examine the anatomy of the fetus. If the second AFP is still high, an ultrasound followed by amniocentesis would be recommended. In most cases, the fetus is normal.

Low AFP Levels

If the AFP level is low, this could indicate Down's syndrome or other chromosomal abnormalities. If this is suspected, a follow-up amniocentesis would then be done to confirm Down's syndrome. However, there are a number of false positives with this test, so you'll still need to follow up with another AFP, ultrasound, and amniocentesis.

False Negatives

Just because your AFP levels are normal doesn't mean that your baby does *not* have a neural tube defect or Down's syndrome. You'll still need ultrasound and possibly amniocentesis if you're in a high-risk group.

Normal Levels

A normal level of AFP means that your baby is most likely normal. In this case, you will not need to follow up with amniocentesis unless you're over 35 or are at a high risk of having a child with Down's syndrome.

The bottom line regarding AFP is that it is not considered "conclusive" in any way; it merely identifies whether your pregnancy is at a higher risk for certain defects, and encourages you to seek other tests to confirm such suspicions.

Amniocentesis

Invented in the 1950s, amniocentesis is always recommended to pregnant women who are over 35 or at high risk of giving birth to a baby with genetic or chromosomal disorders. The procedure involves using an ultrasound to locate a pocket of fluid around the fetus, which makes up the amniotic sac. (The amnion is the inner sac that surrounds the baby and the uterus. This sac contains amniotic fluid, which contains the baby's urine, cells from its skin, and various other chemicals produced by the baby.) Then, a long needle is inserted through the abdomen into the amniotic sac, and amniotic fluid is withdrawn. Most of the time a small amount of local anesthetic is used. You will also need a full bladder for the procedure. The cells in the fluid are then grown in a laboratory and tested for chromosomal abnormalities. The sex of the baby can also be determined through amniocentesis. The results can take between three to four weeks. The procedure is done at 16 weeks to ensure the results are back by 20 weeks. That way, if there *is* a problem, *you* have time to terminate the pregnancy if you wish. Some research centers are performing amniocentesis as early as 14 weeks.

There are risks involved in amniocentesis. Some studies indicate that 1 in 100 normal fetuses is miscarried as a direct result of the procedure, while others report that the risk of miscarriage is as low as 1 in 500. The risk needs to be weighed against the general risk *overall* of a baby born with a deformity: about 4 in 100. Other uncommon side effects of the procedure include a puncture of the placenta, the baby, or the mother's bladder, or an infection or leakage of the amniotic fluid.

What the Test Can Detect:

Most women will have a normal test result. However, it's important to know what this test can find:

- *Chromosomal defects.* These are congenital defects that can cause mental impairment, most commonly Down's syndrome, which is characterized by a flattened face that was once described as "mongoloid." This test is considered very accurate in picking up chromosomal defects.
- *Genetic defects.* Amniocentesis can pick up a long list of metabolic disorders. (Most women would not be tested for a genetic defect unless it was suspected because of a family history or other reason.)
- *The sex of the baby.* This is not determined just for fun but be-

cause it's *imperative* in order to screen for sex-linked diseases such as hemophilia and muscular dystrophy. These diseases are usually passed on to male children by the mother, who acts as a carrier. Chorionic villus sampling (discussed below) can also determine the sex of the child. If you are a carrier of hemophilia but have a female, the baby is presumed out of danger. If you don't want to know the sex of the baby, you should make your preference known before the test is performed.

- *Inherited diseases.* These include Tay-Sachs disease and sickle cell anemia.
- *Open-neural-tube defects.* Spina bifida and anencephaly will be confirmed by this test. Roughly 2 in 1,000 babies are found to have a neural-tube defect. Half them are miscarried; sometimes they are stillborn or die shortly after birth.

Deciding to Have the Test

If you are adamantly opposed to abortion for any reason or believe that your child deserves to live regardless of what kind of genetic disorders are found, then you may feel that there is no reason to have amniocentesis done at all. But even under these circumstances, amniocentesis may be able to prepare you and your family ahead of time and help you make certain decisions regarding delivery. For example, you may decide to refuse a cesarean section if the fetus goes into distress during labor.

The following are legitimate candidates for amniocentesis:

- Women who are clearly at risk of having a child with a genetic disorder or birth defect. These problems include spinal cord defects, missing brain tissue, exposed spinal column, Tay-Sachs disease, and sickle cell anemia.
- Women who are over 35 or at risk for giving birth to a child with a chromosomal disorder known as Down's syndrome, a form of retardation. (Down's syndrome children are now shown to have a much higher capacity to learn and develop

than was once believed. You may need to research your decision to abort a Down's syndrome child.) The majority of all Down's syndrome cases are age-related. At 30, your chances of having a Downs syndrome child are 1 in 885 births; at 35, your chances are 1 in 365; at age 40, the chance goes way up to 1 in 109. This test also picks up other chromosomal abnormalities and would be recommended to someone with a previously affected infant or when either parent has a known chromosomal disorder.

- Women known to be carriers of diseases linked with the female X chromosome, such as one type of muscular dystrophy and hemophilia. These diseases are passed on only to a male child, who in 50% of the cases will develop serious illnesses.
- Women who are diabetic. In the past, amniocentesis was done in the last months of pregnancy to determine the maturity of the baby's lungs. The information was used to determine whether inducing labor was necessary. Yet the tendency these days is to use ultrasound to date pregnancy and then simply monitor the fetus, allowing the labor to occur naturally. There is much less use of amniocentesis in diabetics unless some other condition makes early delivery likely.
- Women who are Rh negative and have produced antibodies that pose a danger to their babies. This is now an uncommon problem. If the baby has been affected, he or she may need an intrauterine transfusion or early delivery, frequently by cesarean section with a transfusion after birth. Cordocentesis, discussed on page 139, may be done instead of amniocentesis.

The following are legitimate reasons to *refuse* amniocentesis:
- You oppose abortion for ethical, moral, or religious reasons.
- You do not wish to risk miscarrying a normal fetus.
- You are comfortable accepting whatever fate is in store for you, and are not able to handle the emotional stress involved with the procedure, regardless of the outcome.

Amnio Questions

There are some risks to the procedure. The safest way to have the procedure done is with the aid of ultrasound and by a doctor experienced with the technique. Most of you who are having amniocentesis will be identified as a high-risk pregnancy from the outset and should be under the care of an obstetrician. However, if you're having the test as a follow-up to a positive AFP, you may *not* be seeing a doctor as familiar with amniocentesis as he or she should be. To be safe, here's what you should ask your doctor before you agree to have it done:

1. Will ultrasound be used to guide me through the procedure? (If not, request that it be used or find another doctor to do it).
2. Will you be doing the procedure yourself? (Sorry, an intern or nurse just won't do. Make sure that the doctor you're seeing is the doctor who does the procedure.)
3. What is this hospital's (or clinic/facility's) rate of miscarriage as a result of amniocentesis? (It shouldn't be higher than 1%.)

Other Available Tests

For now, the "big three" prenatal tests are ultrasound, AFP (the "triple screen"), and amniocentesis. Two more tests may also be used, but neither replace amniocentesis nor ultrasound. They simply indicate further testing, or may be used as a follow-up.

Chorionic Villus Sampling (CVS)

If the idea of amniocentesis bothers you, CVS is considered the amnio alternative. Developed in the late 1980s, this is one of the newest prenatal tests around. It's performed in the *first* trimester, between 8–10 weeks of pregnancy. With the help of ultrasound, a piece of placenta (comprised of small subunits known as chorionic villi) is sampled by inserting a catheter through the vagina and into the uterus. In some cases, due to the location of the placenta, a needle is inserted into the uterus through the abdominal wall. Once you're beyond 11 weeks, the window for the test closes, because amniocentesis becomes available at 13 weeks, which can pick up more problems.

CVS can detect the same chromosomal defects as amniocentesis, but it cannot diagnose open-neural-tube defects. Depending upon the type of analysis you need, results may be available within 24 hours or can take up to two weeks. Some doctors report that results can take as long as four weeks. However, you will need to have a serum AFP done at 15–16 weeks if you go the CVS route.

There are risks. First, CVS carries a slightly higher risk of miscarriage than amniocentesis. Your risk for miscarriage with CVS increases to between 2% and 4% over the natural risk for miscarriage during this trimester: 1 in 6 pregnancies. Studies suggest that if the test is performed before 10 weeks, there can be an increased risk of fetal limb developmental problems.

It is also more difficult to interpret the results of CVS. Occasionally, chromosome variants or mixtures of cell types make interpretation difficult. In these cases, a blood sample might be needed from both parents to see if there really is a problem.

Why have this test?

If you're in a high-risk group for a chromosomal problem, this test can detect it very early, and you can have a first-trimester abortion. This is all fine in theory, but because the test results can sometimes be difficult to interpret, the decision to abort should be made only after consulting with a genetic counselor. If your CVS is normal, you will follow it up with AFP, ultrasound, and possibly amniocentesis. If you're going to terminate the pregnancy, you must be sure that a problem exists.

Cordocentesis

Also known as *cord blood sampling* or *percutaneous umbilical blood sampling*

(PUBS), cordocentesis can sample some of the fetus's blood. This test is done in the second half of the pregnancy *usually when a fetal abnormality has already been detected via ultrasound*. Genetic studies are done to confirm or even pinpoint a problem. You also can get the results very quickly, in about 48 hours, so that you can make the proper decision about whether to terminate the pregnancy. This test is done by using ultrasound to identify the area where the umbilical cord inserts into the placenta. You'll receive a local anesthetic, and a small amount of fetal blood is withdrawn with a long, fine needle. After the procedure, the fetal heart rate will need to be observed for several minutes.

The risk is considered higher than with amniocentesis. There may be signs of immediate fetal distress or premature labor. Again, this test is done only if a problem has already been identified. The procedure can also be used for intrauterine transfusion in pregnancies affected by Rh incompatibility.

In the Near Future

As with any technology, new prenatal tests are being developed all the time. The latest prenatal test on the drawing board is the use of *magnetic resonance imaging (MRI)*. MRI can be used to diagnose all kinds of health problems, such as heart disease, cancer, multiple sclerosis, and some birth defects in a developing fetus.

How MRI works

This technology uses large magnets to build a video picture. Since much of your body is made up of water and hydrogen atoms, when placed in a magnetic field and surrounded by radiowaves, the hydrogen atoms are transformed into a type of energy that releases a faint radio signal. This signal is then translated by a computer into an image. Tissue containing more water, such as fatty tissue, will look different than bone, which contains very little water. Used in obstetrics, MRI can give us images of the developing fetus, and can identify structural problems. MRI is not used very much yet because:

- It's very expensive and requires specially equipped rooms.
- There are concerns that MRI can harm a developing fetus.

However, once MRI is tested and proved to pose no risks to the fetus, it may become just as standard a prenatal test as ultrasound. To date, however, ultrasound is considered far superior in terms of cost, convenience, and technology.

Terminating the Pregnancy

The purpose of prenatal testing is to tell you whether your baby will be "normal." Obviously, most women will be anxious about the results and will want to be comforted by the good news that all is well. However, bear in mind that there are countless *physical* deformities that are correctable with surgery; these options should be discussed with a neonatal specialist and factored into your decision. If amniocentesis confirms Down's syndrome or another chromosomal abnormality, you'll need to discuss with your doctor *exactly* how your baby will be affected. Attitudes toward persons with Down's syndrome are changing, and many families choose to welcome these children with their special needs, which can include mild to moderate retardation and physical and medical problems. For other families, abortion might be the best choice. Other chromosomal abnormalities cause conditions that are not compatible with life. Being aware of the problem ahead of time can prepare you for the likelihood of stillbirth or neonatal death. In these cases, many parents consider pregnancy termination (even though they would not in other circumstances). It's also important to note that if the decision is made to allow the pregnancy to continue, a futile cesarean for distress of the fetus during labor may be avoided.

Whatever you decide, remember that the decision to abort or *not* to abort is a personal and private choice that has more to do with your civil rights as an individual than it does with your health.

The Therapeutic Abortion

While I sincerely hope that you will not *need* to read the following, statistics show that many of you are older and are at greater risk of having pregnancies with fetal abnormalities. That means that some of you *will* make the decision to terminate your pregnancy. As I stated in the introduction, this book is designed to give you the information you need for the duration of your pregnancy. While this *is* a pregnancy book, the termination of a pregnancy is an obstetrical fact of life in the mid-1990s.

Abortion is far from a dirty word. Medically, the word *abortion* simply refers to pregnancy loss before the 28th week. This may be either a *spontaneous abortion,* also known as miscarriage (which includes *complete, missed,* or *incomplete abortion,* discussed in chapter 3), or a *therapeutic abortion (TA),* defined as "a deliberate termination of pregnancy for medical or social reasons."

If you decide to terminate the pregnancy, the surgical abortion procedure you undergo will depend on whether you're in your first or second trimester of pregnancy. This section covers abortions in the second trimester, which is where you'll be in your pregnancy when you make your decision to terminate. After the pregnancy has progressed beyond a certain number of weeks in the second trimester (usually 24 weeks, but the legal limit varies, you will *not* be able to elect to terminate the pregnancy legally. All women in North America can expect to have a legal abortion *up until at least their 20th week of pregnancy.* This is why getting your prenatal tests done as early as possible is imperative.

In some cases, terminating your pregnancy may be suggested to you by your obstetrics practitioner. There are two basic reasons:

- When continuing the pregnancy endangers your life. You may have developed a heart condition or a severe illness during the pregnancy, or you may have discovered that you are HIV positive and now have to choose between your life and that of the unborn child.
- When the fetus is malformed or will be born with an inevitable genetic/chromosomal deformity. Again, some of these

problems are salvageable with surgery, some problems may be acceptable to you, and others may mean an unhappy future for all concerned. If your financial resources are limited, bear in mind that neonatal care and treatment in the Unite States is extremely expensive.

Who should not consider an abortion for defective pregnancy?

Abortion is not the definitive solution for every unwanted pregnancy. That's why it's important to explore options to abortion first to make sure that an abortion is what you *really* want. In general, there are two groups who may not benefit from an abortion:

1. *Women who are morally or ethically opposed to abortion.* For example, even though you *know* you're carrying a child that is malformed, you may not be able to go through with terminating the pregnancy. The psychological trauma to you may be lessened by giving birth to the child and letting fate decide the outcome.

2. *Women who don't feel informed enough about their options.* Have you considered adoption? Or looked into social programs that might support your special needs child? Have you researched your decision to abort? Are you familiar with what the procedure entails? Have you explored all other solutions?

Abortion in the second trimester

Until about five years ago, women who had abortions done beyond 16 weeks were subjected to a horrible procedure known as *amnioinduction,* or induction abortion or miscarriage. This procedure entailed checking into a hospital, having your obstetrics practitioner insert a needle into your abdomen, and injecting a miscarriage-inducing solution into the amniotic sac (usually a saline solution), which killed the fetus by poisoning it. You were required to wait about 24 hours for labor to set in, and then you *literally went into labor* (discussed in chapter 7) *and gave birth to the dead fetus.* This is a procedure that has perhaps fueled the pro-life activists more than any other. Worse, because an amnioinduction procedure involves childbirth, there are numerous complications involved as well.

In 1995, no woman living *anywhere* in North America needs to subject herself to an amnioinduction procedure. A far safer, cheaper, shorter, and less traumatic *D & E* procedure *(dilatation and evacuation)* is now the standard second-trimester procedure performed. *And it can be done right up until the 24th week of pregnancy.* The only reason amnioinduction still exists as a procedure at all is because there aren't enough doctors in North America trained to do a D & E procedure. If you live in a large city that has plenty of excellent hospitals and facilities, you won't have any trouble getting a D & E in the second trimester. If you live in an under-populated area, ask your gynecologist or primary care physician for the name of a doctor or clinic that does second trimester D & Es. If this fails, call either the National Abortion Federation or the Planned Parenthood Federation of America. Tell them that you need to have a second trimester D & E procedure done, let them know how far along you are in the pregnancy, and make it clear that you're interested *only* in clinics advanced or large enough to perform this procedure. Once you have a referral, phone ahead to the clinic to confirm that they do the procedure, make an appointment, and *travel* to that clinic (probably located in a larger city) to get the D & E done. *The expense of an amnioinduction procedure is equal to, if not more than, a roundtrip bus or train fare and the cost of a D & E procedure.* If anyone tries to convince you that a D & E procedure is not appropriate this late or that it involves more complications, don't believe them. This is just not true! Amnioinduction is an archaic and cruel procedure that has been abandoned by skilled obstetrics practitioners.

What to expect in a D & E procedure

First, you'll need to have your cervix dilated prior to the procedure. You'll have a seaweed root called *laminaria* or a similar synthetic dilator inserted into your cervical opening 24 hours before the procedure. After insertion, you'll be sent home and will report back to the hospital the next day for the procedure. Depending on how well your cervix is dilated from the first laminaria, you may need to have additional laminaria inserted, and hence, wait longer to have the procedure.

Fresh laminaria will be inserted into your cervical opening once you're dilated enough, and the doctor will administer a local anesthetic. A tube will then be inserted into your cervical opening and attached to a vacuum pump, through which the contents of the uterus are suctioned out. Forceps may also be used to help retrieve larger pieces of fetal tissue. You'll feel cramping as the uterus contracts during the procedure. A standard D & C procedure will then be done, after which it's all over. This entire procedure takes about 20 minutes at the most. (Some sources estimate as little as 10 minutes and others say as long as 45 minutes.)

The aftereffects

Most women will experience some irregular bleeding, cramping, or spotting for about two weeks. Some women will continue to experience menstrual-like cramping and bleeding for as long as six weeks afterward. Taking anti-inflammatory medication is helpful in this case.

You might experience feelings of depression following the abortion, which stem from normal grief following the abortion and are not abnormal. It's important to seek post-abortion counseling with a counselor from the clinic. Review the "Postpartum Depression" section in chapter 10. You'll probably experience feelings that range from the blues to bona fide depression. If these feelings don't pass within a couple of weeks, you may need longer-term therapy to fully recover emotionally.

You'll also need to follow certain hygiene guidelines after the procedure, outlined in chapter 8. You should refrain from sexual intercourse until your cervix has resumed its normal size.

Your period will return about 4–6 weeks after the procedure. Because your lining has been removed and your body is rebalancing its hormones, it will take that long for your menstrual cycle to get back on track. However, you *can* get pregnant immediately after an abortion.

If you experience any hemorrhaging or heavy bleeding, you'll need to see your doctor as soon as possible. There are treatments available that will control the bleeding, which is usually caused at this stage by retained placental tissue in the uterus.

If all goes well with your prenatal tests, and your pregnancy progresses as planned, your discomfort increases while the risk of something going wrong increases as well. At the same time, preparing for labor and delivery becomes serious business. Onward . . . or downward . . . it all depends on your perspective.

6

T3 Health (Trimester 3)

Once you've made it past all those prenatal tests and are in the home stretch, you'll begin preparing for labor and childbirth. Childbirth education classes are discussed in this chapter, while labor and delivery are discussed separately in chapter 7. You'll also begin to feel as though you've been pregnant forever. "Wait" now seems to be more important than weight.

Unfortunately, as the time of childbirth draws near, the risk of complications increases. Premature labor and delivery, as well as health complications that warrant being induced or having a cesarean section, will surface at this stage.

The unique problems with multiple births and postmature deliveries are also discussed, as well as the phenomenon known as false labor. I've included another section on sex, which gets more challenging and tricky as you become larger. (Also, review the sex section in chapter 4.) Finally, I've provided a section on antepartum fetal testing. Everything about the "waiting game"—trimester 3—is here.

How Does It Feel?

In chapters 3 and 4, I've provided an alphabetical breakdown of assorted pregnancy discomforts. The list in chapter 4 actually covers all of the discomforts you may be experiencing right now, but some symptoms will become more intense, while others will lessen.

By this stage your uterus has probably become very large and very hard. The baby's movements are visible, and, if you haven't already, you'll begin to experience the Braxton Hicks contractions, discussed in chapter 4. You'll feel periodic tightening in the uterus. There will also be an increase in urinary pressure, and you'll need to urinate more frequently, as you did in the first trimester.

You'll also experience more shortness of breath as the baby presses on your diaphragm. Once the baby moves down more into your pelvis in the last month or so, this will ease off. This is known as lightening because you may actually feel much lighter as a result (but don't count on it).

Sleeping will become more difficult. First, depending on your size, you may not be able to find a comfortable sleeping position. As a result, you'll be tossing and turning all night. Second, you'll become more anxious and excited about the baby and may not be able stop your mind from racing in a hundred different directions. All this boils down to one word: fatigue. Some women find adjustable beds helpful. You can rent one for this last period.

Because you'll have gained an additional 10–15 pounds in this trimester alone, you'll become uncoordinated, feel awkward, and may experience backaches and leg pains. The most common back pain at this stage is lower back pain; your expanding uterus is changing your posture, which is straining your back. The only real remedy available is changing your position. You can consult either your own doctor or a chiropractor about sitting and standing positions that will put less pressure on your back. Lying down with your feet elevated may also help to alleviate the strain. Before you relieve a sore back with ice or hot baths, however, it's important to consult your doctor; sometimes applying heat is the worst thing you can do, and can aggravate the situation. As for ice, it's only effective in short intervals (10 minutes on/10 minutes off). Hormonal changes in your body can also cause your hip, groin, and tailbone to separate a little, which will hurt. Again, lying down and elevating your feet is just about the only thing you can do. You may also experience a type of joint looseness caused by progesterone, which relaxes certain muscles and prepares your body for labor. There is a very good reason for all this weight gain. Between weeks 33 and 40 (where your due date should fall), your baby gains more than half of its birth weight. This weight is necessary for the baby to survive outside of the uterus.

Finally, all the second trimester health problems you may have developed will persist: edema, venous changes, autoimmune disorders, and so on. And believe it or not, some women still suffer from morning sickness at this stage! By now you'll have learned to live with these changes, but may need to consult with your doctor if symptoms become really uncomfortable.

The bottom line is that by this stage you will be tired of the pregnancy. You'll be tired of hemorrhoids or any other side effects you're experiencing, tired of having to pee every five minutes, tired of all your maternity clothes, tired of your weight and size, and tired of WAITING! These feelings of wanting to "get it over with" are common, normal, and healthy.

Five Easy Symptoms that Spell H-E-A-L-T-H-Y

As unpleasant as all these discomforts may be, there are five key symptoms at this stage that are important signs of fetal health and well-being. The absence of any one of these symptoms should be noted and reported to your doctor.

1. Fetal movement. Kicking is an excellent sign that will undoubtedly keep you up at night. You should be recording this fetal movement on a "kick chart" that your doctor should have supplied you with by this stage. *Warning: If you notice the absence*

*of any fetal movement in a 12-hour period, notify your doctor imme-
diately. This is a sign that the baby may be in trouble.*

2. Breathlessness. If you're short of breath GOOD! You should be, since your lungs need to work twice as hard to supply both you and the baby with oxygen. In addition, the baby should be large enough now that it is pressing up against your lungs, making you feel short of breath. Basically, each time you gasp for air, your baby is getting just the right amount at your expense. Normally, breathlessness isn't a problem unless you're asthmatic. Asthma is discussed briefly in chapter 2.

3. Frequent urination to the point of slight incontinence. It may be maddening to be "chained" to a toilet, but wanting to urinate every five minutes or so means that your baby is traveling down toward your vagina and getting into position. This is a good sign. What's happening is that not only is the baby large enough that it's pressing down on your bladder (and other internal organs), but progesterone is smoothing out and relaxing your muscles to prepare you for labor, enabling your body to make the stretch. Normally, when you urinate, your muscles go into a relaxed mode. But when you're pregnant, they're in a constant state of relaxation, which will make you want to urinate . . . RIGHT NOW! This is normal and nothing to worry about, and it may even result in some involuntary leakage of urine. This symptom means that the head is in the right place and your baby's weight and size are appropriate for this stage.

4. Braxton Hicks contractions. Discussed above and in chapter 4, these contractions are sometimes mistaken for labor but are very different from labor contractions. (If you're carrying twins, you may not be able to feel these. See below.) Basically, these feel as though your abdominal area suddenly tightens up and then relaxes. These contractions start anywhere in the second or early third trimester and get more intense as you move toward your due date. By now the tightening will last about 20

seconds at the most. Labor contractions, however, are much stronger and last at least 40 seconds.

5. Lightening: engagement of the head. This is when the baby's head drops down slightly into the upper part of the pelvis, at last releasing your lungs from its grip. Until now your uterus has been expanding upward toward your lungs to accommodate the baby's size. But by the 36th week or so, your uterus expands more to prepare for labor and delivery, giving your baby more headroom! This extra space allows the head to drop down a little, relieving your upper body of all the pressure it's been feeling. The term lightening has been coined *not* because you'll lose weight, but because you'll feel as though a weight has been lifted off your chest. In other words, you'll be breathing easier as a result of this drop.

The Multiple Waiting Game

The rules of the waiting game are a little different for women with multiple-birth pregnancies. First of all, you should expect to deliver prematurely. In fact, premature births occur 10 times more often with multiple births than with single births. And, as mentioned in chapter 2, the more fetuses you're carrying, the shorter your gestation period. Currently, about 50% of all twins and 75% of all triplets are born before the 37th week. The most common cause of premature birth in multiple births is a premature dilation of the cervix, caused by a thinning out of the cervix prior to 36 weeks. No one really knows why this happens, but it may likely be caused by basic physics: overstuff a paper bag, and it's going to break; overstuff a uterus, and it's going to break, sooner than later. For most women, the cervix was designed to hold one baby securely, not two or more. Therefore, because of the increased incidence in cervical effacement (the thinning out of the cervix) in multiple births, the cervix should be routinely checked in a pelvic exam performed during a routine prenatal visit.

Another problem with multiple pregnancies in this trimester is that you may not be able to detect any contractions at all, because your uterus is stretched out to the maximum tautness. This also means that you may not be able to feel Braxton Hicks contractions. Finally, you may be confusing fetal movement with contractions. The best thing you can do if you're not sure about whether labor has begun is to first review the premature labor section below for all the possible signs and symptoms of labor (some of which are vague). Then, see your doctor immediately and ask him or her to check your cervix for signs of dilation. A dilated cervix means you're about to go into or are already in labor. Women who have given birth to twins report a range of odd labor experiences, ranging from feeling like they had "just gas" to "just lower back pains" to "just feeling funny."

Your Last-Minute Tune-Up

As discussed in chapter 4, unless you're a high-risk pregnancy (see chapter 2), your prenatal exams will be fairly routine until about the eighth month of pregnancy. By this point, you'll go for a prenatal exam roughly every two weeks, and then graduate to weekly exams by the last month until you deliver. You can also expect to have a sort of last minute tune-up as your doctor checks for any signs of hypertension, toxemia, protein, or sugar in your urine. All of these conditions are discussed in chapter 2. And, of course, you'll be weighed. You'll need to weigh enough to nourish the child in this last stage, but you'll need to make sure your weight doesn't predispose you to other health problems such as hypertension or diabetes. If your doctor does find signs that you may have developed one of these problems, he or she will most likely follow up with an ultrasound scan to see if the baby is growing at the right rate (not too large and not too small for its age). Your doctor may also want to monitor your baby's heartbeat with a fetal heart monitor, which can help to anticipate potential problems during delivery.

As discussed in chapter 5, even if the pregnancy is progressing at a perfectly normal rate, you may need to have a second ultrasound scan done in the last month or so to check the baby's "lie," its position. Basically, your doctor needs to know whether the baby is in the optimum position for delivery. For example, is the baby in the correct position for a vaginal delivery? (Is it "head first" or breech?) The baby can actually be turned around in some instances if it's not in a good position, but it's tricky and not often attempted. This is discussed more fully below.

How to Tell a "Lie"

The "lie" refers to your baby's position. There are several different positions that will work; there are also several positions that will make vaginal delivery difficult. The position of the baby can most often be determined by your doctor just feeling your abdomen by hand. If there's any questions about the lie, it can be resolved through ultrasound. As stated above, your second ultrasound will confirm whether your baby's head is in the correct position for a vaginal delivery. If your baby's head is looking toward heaven and the feet are toward your vagina, this is known as the breech position. This is not a great position to be in, but it's common for the baby to turn itself back to the correct position, with its head down toward your vagina, between the 32nd week and your due date. It's also possible for your doctor to turn the baby, but many doctors prefer not to because of the risk of interfering with the placenta or triggering premature labor. In fact only about 3% of all deliveries are breech.

Whether your baby is in the breech position or correct position for birth, a vaginal delivery can be done as long as the baby is in a longitudinal lie (vertical). Longitudinal lies vary in about nine different positions. With its head in the correct position; the baby's left or right ear may be facing you; its back may face you, tilted to the left or right; its front may face you, or, rarely but interestingly, it may have its head thrown back and have its face delivered first in a kind of nose-dive position (called a face presentation).

In the breech position, the baby's legs may be crossed or extended upward into a sitting position (so the baby is in a V-shape), making for a buttocks-first delivery; the feet may dangle down, or sometimes the knees are bent and will be delivered first.

A vaginal delivery is not possible if your baby is in a transverse lie (horizontal). This means that either its head or feet is facing your appendix instead of your vagina! In this case, a cesarean delivery will be the only way to safely deliver the baby. Turning the baby, again, may be attempted in rare instances, but don't count on it.

What About Sex?

By this stage, most women really don't feel all that sexy. Your hormonal balance has shifted, and your sex drive may have drastically diminished. On top of this, you will feel large and awkward and may not feel comfortable in any sexual intercourse position. If you have hemorrhoids, you'll likely be very uncomfortable and will not be up to having too much sex.

Regardless of how uninterested you may be, your partner may likely be climbing the walls by this point. What many couples do at this stage is compromise: You bring him to orgasm manually or orally; he gives you back rubs and foot massages and goes out in the middle of the night to find you chocolate chip cookie dough ice cream, or whatever. It's important not to put your partner in the position of "begging" for sexual relief or make him feel like a "pervert" because he's aroused. As awkward as you may feel, he may find your pregnant shape extremely arousing, particularly your breasts. Unless you're communicating about your sexual needs, serious relationship problems can arise out of these seemingly trivial issues, and wind up dividing you. The last thing you need when you're caring for a newborn is a divisive relationship with your partner. Be patient with one another and exchange favors.

If you do feel in the mood, your best bet is the "spoon position" (side by side, his penis facing your buttocks). This allows you and your belly to rest comfortably on the bed, eliminating the need to exert yourself too much. Will sexual stimulation trigger labor prematurely? It depends. For a normal, routine pregnancy, multiple orgasms and vigorous nipple stimulation should not trigger labor. If, however, you're having twins or are experiencing other health problems with your pregnancy, nipple stimulation and orgasm may trigger labor prematurely. Again, frankly discuss your sexual activity with your doctor and find out if there are any boundaries he or she suggests you don't cross.

If you're close to your due date and don't mind tempting labor, try bringing yourself to orgasm and stimulating your nipples (either manually or with a little help from your partner). Sex after childbirth is discussed in chapter 8.

Childbirth 101: Starting Classes

Thirty years ago it was unheard of for an expectant couple to take a class in childbirth. Today it's unheard of for an expectant couple *not* to experience at least one such class. Childbirth classes usually begin when you're about eight weeks away from labor—anywhere from your 30th to 32nd week.

The classes usually explain coaching, show films, and discuss all kinds of labor and delivery scenarios, including what to do in emergency situations, as discussed below. Childbirth classes are definitely one of the best ways to prepare yourself and your partner for labor and delivery. However, many women find that these classes are a joke. This can happen if you have a poor instructor or if the class has a weak curriculum, teaching you nothing that you don't already know from articles, magazines, or other books. You should also make sure that the class is teaching you the kind of childbirth method you intend to use. If you're not interested in Lamaze, for example, don't take a Lamaze class.

To avoid bad classes, make sure you go to a class that your practitioner or midwife personally recommends, or even one that is provided at your birthing facility. Make sure the instructor is qualified and certified by the Childbirth Education Association, and isn't just the "mother of six." Just because the instructor has children doesn't guarantee that she can teach! She (or even he) needs to have teaching and communication skills, and some medical training (nurse, midwife, etc.). Before you sign up, you can sit in on some classes to test out various centers or instructors.

Essentially, there are three basic "methods" out there: Grantly Dick-Read, Lamaze, and Bradley, all named after the practitioners who invented various techniques for breathing, working with pain, and teaching fathers to be coaches and active participants in the labor process. Other classes are more healthcare oriented, borrowing techniques from all three methods, tailoring your class to the newest technology and information available and, if given by your birthing facility, tailoring information specifically to it.

General Curriculum Guidelines

It doesn't matter whether your class is taught by a Lamaze purist or a down-to-earth midwife. What does matter is whether you're getting the appropriate information. Your course curriculum should include:

- Information on prenatal care and hygiene. If you've read the previous chapters, this information will feel like a summer rerun, but it's important to go over this material as often as you can.
- Fetal development throughout each stage of the pregnancy. See appendix B for recommended books on this area.
- The changes your body experiences as the pregnancy progresses. Again, this material will be a rerun, but your class should contain it nevertheless.
- Warning signs at various stages of the pregnancy, and emergency procedures for each problem. This information is imperative. You can never review emergency procedures too often.
- Labor 101. Your class should cover all three stages of labor and include breathing techniques, coaching techniques, pain relief, and information about episiotomies.
- Problems that warrant being induced or having a cesarean section. You should be totally prepared for situations that may call for cesareans or being induced.

- Breastfeeding or bottle-feeding? All the pitfalls and benefits of each decision should be presented, covering the appropriate feeding techniques, positioning, and bras you'll need. Nipple care and possible nipple infections should be discussed as well. (See chapter 9 for this material.)
- Baby tools. All the baby "stuff" you need to buy, such as clothing, furniture, car seats. (In Canada, hospitals will not release a newborn unless the parents have a proper car seat in their vehicle, installed in accordance with government specifications.)
- Baby lessons. You should learn how to hold, change, and bathe your baby.
- A tour of your birthing facility. If your class is at your birthing facility, you'll be given a tour of the maternity ward and labor ward and see all the technological equipment (fetal monitoring equipment) that will be used. If your class is at a separate center, book your tour separately with your hospital or birthing facility and take it "after class."
- Health and contraception after childbirth. This information is also covered in chapter 8.

Things that Can Go Wrong

This time, most of the problems that occur are related to complications that cause premature labor and delivery, postmaturity, and complications that may necessitate being induced or delivered by cesarean section.

Other problems revolve around your general health, which in turn could affect the baby's health. Gestational diabetes, gestational hypertension, and toxemia (preeclampsia or eclampsia) are all health hazards that can carry nasty consequences, resulting in stillbirth or premature birth. This is why a technologically advanced birthing facility is so important.

Many of these problems are expertly and speedily dealt with when they come up to ensure both your own and your baby's health.

Premature Labor and Delivery

There's no such thing as miscarriage at this stage. When you miscarry in late pregnancy, you graduate to premature labor. This means that for a variety of reasons, your body isn't able to carry full term and begins to give birth. Some reasons for premature labor at this stage include infections (STDs or others), hypertension, drugs and smoking, placental problems (see below), uterine structural problems, and cervical incompetence. However, most cases of premature labor have unknown causes. Premature labor is no different than any other labor; it just happens before the baby is as physically able to exist in the outside world as it is at nine months. North American obstetricians consider premature labor to be one of the biggest problems. Neonatal technology is very expensive (paid for in Canada by universal health care). Currently, 6–8% of all babies are born prematurely, which accounts for 75% of all neonatal deaths.

Who will deliver prematurely?

Again, most women who deliver prematurely are not in a high-risk group for preterm labor. Nevertheless, it's important to know who's statistically more at risk for preterm labor:

- women with a history of preterm labor;
- women carrying multiple fetuses;
- women who have had abdominal surgery during pregnancy (fibroid surgery, cysts removed, and so on);
- women with a history of two second trimester miscarriages or therapeutic abortions;
- women with a cervix less than 1 centimeter long;
- women whose cervix is dilated more than 1 centimeter;
- women who are DES daughters (see chapter 2);
- women who have ever had a cone biopsy done of their cervix;
- women with an incompetent cervix (discussed in chapter 4);

- women with an irritable uterus;
- women who have excessive amniotic fluid (polyhydramnios); and
- women with a double uterus.

Symptoms of premature labor

Classic symptoms of premature labor are clear, watery, mucusy, or bloody vaginal discharge, a tightening of the uterus, a lower backache that feels a little different than usual, and pressure in the pelvis area.

But there are other symptoms of premature labor you might not recognize. These include contractions that occur at regular intervals of 15 minutes or less; menstrual-like cramps that are either rhythmic or continuous; a rhythmic pressure that seems to bounce off your thighs; gas pains, digestive problems, or diarrhea; and a vague lower backache that feels like a "normal" backache. Finally, an intuitive sense that something doesn't "feel right" in conjunction with a vague symptom may also be sign that you're in labor.

Can you stop premature labor once it starts?

Sometimes. Drinking several glasses of water will often prevent labor from progressing. If you're in a hospital, intravenous fluids may be used to achieve the same results. The water helps prevent falling blood volume and contractions from taking place. If drinking water at home doesn't seem to help, get yourself to a hospital as soon as possible.

Medications

Certain medications can be used to postpone labor, however, they can be used only if your cervix is intact (not dilated beyond 3 centimeters and not thinned out, or effaced). These are known as tocolytic drugs and help to suppress uterine contractions. These drugs must always be first administered in a hospital or proper birthing facility. For the most part, tocolytic medications have generally been used safely since the 1970s. The most commonly prescribed drugs are *ritodrine* (Yutopar) and *terbutaline* (Brethine). Ritodrine was approved by the FDA in 1988, and terbutaline has not yet been approved, but works by the same method, and is cheaper. In this case, the manufacturer has not yet applied for FDA approval. Both drugs carry side effects, including increased heart rate, palpitations, tremors, anxiety, and low blood pressure. Ritodrine can cause pulmonary congestion, so it's not a good idea for asthmatics. The main idea behind tocolytic drugs is to postpone labor. If labor is prevented, it's possible to continue to take these medications orally at home.

Who should not take these drugs?

If you have the following conditions, your labor should not be inhibited, and hence, you won't be offered any tocolytic medications.
- have severe gestational hypertension;
- have severe placental problems (see below);
- have an infection of the amniotic fluid; or
- are carrying a child with severe defects or a child who has died in utero.

You should question your doctor about taking these drugs if you:
- have chronic but mild hypertension;
- have mild placental abnormalities;
- have cardiac disease;
- are hyperthyroid (from Graves' disease, for example);
- are diabetic; or
- have a dilated cervix.

Depending on your condition, you may still be able to take these medications safely under this second set of conditions if, for example, premature labor is more hazardous to you and your baby than preventing labor.

Generally, if you're more than 35 weeks pregnant, your baby's lungs are mature, your cervix is 4 centimeters dilated or more, and your amniotic sac has broken (discussed in chapter 7), your doctor will not interfere with labor and you'll deliver.

Placental Problems

As mentioned above, placental problems are often the culprits behind premature labor. Bleeding is usually the first symptom of a placenta problem.

Low-lying placenta, or placenta previa

One in every 200 pregnancies will experience this. This simply refers to the position of the placenta and means that it is a little too low, near the mouth of the uterus, and may cover the cervix. The placenta in this case is in fine form. It's just in the wrong position. The bleeding is bright red and painless. It starts out suddenly and can be triggered by coughing, straining, or sexual intercourse (see section above and chapter 4). This condition is diagnosed via ultrasound. If it happens in the second trimester, the placenta may "move" away from the cervix by late pregnancy and, in a way, correct itself.

Treatment may include a combination of bed rest, a variety of vitamin or dietary supplements, hospitalization for bed rest and monitoring, and even transfusions. Sometimes the pregnancy is kept going until about the 36th week. At that point you'll be delivered by cesarean, and the baby will be kept in a neonatal wing until it is strong enough to survive at home. In the worst case scenario, a very premature delivery may be necessary.

Premature separation of the placenta, or abruptio placenta

One in four cases of mid-to-late pregnancy bleeding is caused by abrupto placenta, which means that the placenta has separated itself prematurely from the uterus. One in every 50–80 pregnancies will develop this problem. In 90% of the cases, mother and baby are fine. The bleeding is like a light or even heavy menstrual flow and may contain clots or cause cramping or mild cramps or pain in the abdomen. In more severe cases, bleeding is heavy, which could cause fetal death and maternal blood problems. Ultrasound may be helpful in diagnosis. Cocaine use during pregnancy can cause the separation. The remedy is bed rest and careful monitoring. If the fetus is in distress (see chapter 7), induced labor and premature delivery is necessary. In many cases, you go into spontaneous labor when you have this problem. In this case, it's wise not to stop labor with any medications. Treatment really depends on a few things: the degree of separation (is it partial or total separation?); the severity of the bleeding (heavy or mild); and so on. Total separation will warrant an emergency cesarean section, while partial separation may warrant just being monitored for a while and then being induced and delivering vaginally.

Absence of Fetal Movement

In addition to symptoms of labor, warning signs at this stage have to do with an absence of fetal movement. If you've felt no movement for more than 12 hours, you should contact your doctor immediately and find out what's wrong. Often, the fetus is just sleeping, but do not take any chances. One way around "is it alive or not?"—which all mothers will go through is to purchase an actual stethoscope earlier on in the pregnancy, and have your doctor show you and your partner how to use it and what to listen for. Remember, 30 years ago, this was the only kind of prenatal "monitoring" that was done. You'll want to be able to check for the heartbeat and observe any abnormalities.

Stillbirth

Stillbirth is pretty rare these days, particularly since facilities are equipped with advanced fetal monitoring equipment. When a fetus dies in the womb, its oxygen supply is somehow cut off. During a normal labor and delivery, cord complications are anticipated, and the delivery staff is prepared for any number of problems. Women are monitored for this, and, if it does happen, an emergency cesarean is done.

If the amniotic environment becomes hostile for any reason, labor is induced to prevent a potential stillbirth. This can happen because of leakage of amniotic fluid, malfunction of the placenta, an overdue pregnancy, toxemia, and a host of other health problems.

Sometimes a perfectly healthy baby, born alive, may have problems when the cord is cut, but its lungs or heart fails to oxygenate its system. In a hospital setting, the baby would be given oxygen immediately and speedily resuscitated.

The first scenario can happen at some point in the second or third trimester, well before labor complications are even a consideration. Should you experience a stillbirth, you will need to give birth to that fetus. Labor is usually induced as soon as the tragedy is confirmed. You will definitely need to seek out counseling and must expect to properly grieve for that child. You might also find it helpful to have an autopsy conducted to find out exactly what happened. Naming the child and properly burying or cremating it is the normal practice. Stillbirth is considered one of the most difficult and traumatic experiences a woman will ever go through. You will need to surround yourself with supportive people and come to terms with the loss before you can try to conceive again. Religious clergy may be very helpful to you during these times.

False Labor

This is a common problem that has more to do with misinformation and natural anxiety than physiology. Most women go into false labor because they mistake Braxton Hicks contractions for the real thing. This is understandable, particularly if this is your first baby. To further complicate the issue, Braxton Hicks contractions can become more intense as the pregnancy progresses, to point of being painful. Many women mistake the pain for a sure sign of labor. Here's a quick checklist that explains the differences between Braxton Hicks contractions and true labor contractions:

- Braxton Hicks contractions are irregular rather than rhythmic.
- Braxton Hicks contractions are shorter, lasting 30 seconds at the most, while labor contractions last at least 40 seconds.
- Your cervix does not dilate with Braxton Hicks contractions in any way, something that always accompanies true labor contractions.

If you're not sure . . . .

Take a walk. Walking will help true labor progress, and lessen the frequency of false labor pains. Call your doctor and report your symptoms. He or she may be able to tell you over the phone that you are not in labor or may want to check your cervix for signs of dilation. A typical scenario is being anxious, feeling certain that "this is it," and going to the hospital only to find that the contractions have become very irregular and your cervix isn't dilated. You then go home to wait some more. This is a universal third-trimester beef.

Still Waiting: The Postmature Baby

You're still reading this chapter? You're 41 weeks pregnant? Your due date has come and gone? Relax and join the club: about 8–11% of all pregnancies extend beyond the typical 40-week gestation period.

There are a few reasons why your big day may not have arrived yet. First, the date of your last menstrual period may have been miscalculated, which will mean that your due date was miscalculated as well. Miscalculations are common in women who have irregular menstrual cycles or who were on oral contraception prior to the pregnancy. Second, if you've previously given birth to a post-mature baby, you're statistically more likely to repeat your experience.

The problem with a postterm pregnancy is that you'll want to prevent a condition known as *postmaturity*, where the placenta basically wears out, no longer able to nourish the fetus. In a sense, the fetus in this case overstays its welcome eating itself out of house and home. When this happens, the baby stops growing and may actually start to waste away, losing weight and getting thinner and weaker. The womb, meanwhile, becomes a hostile environment. At 43 weeks, the baby's life becomes 5 times riskier in the womb than outside, while at 44 weeks the baby's life becomes 7 times riskier in the womb than outside. Because of this, many postterm pregnancies are induced after being monitored for 2 weeks. If you're past 2 weeks, and the baby is healthy and vigorous, and postmaturity has not set in, your doctor may in fact do nothing and wait a little longer until natural labor sets in.

Antepartum Fetal Testing: Is the Fetus Stressed Out?

There are several medical conditions that may warrant what's known as antepartum fetal testing. This is different than prenatal testing in that you're looking for placental problems or amniotic fluid problems that may trigger fetal distress (discussed in chapter 7). Antepartum testing consists of a group of tests that may vary from woman to woman, and depends on how healthy you and the fetus are.

The Non-stress Test

Here, an electronic fetal monitor is used to record the fetal heart rate and contractions (if they're there). In addition, the mother, nurse, or other observer is asked to record any fetal movement felt. In a normal test (called a reactive test), the fetal heartrate increases when the baby moves. In an abnormal test (called a nonreactive test), there is no increase in the fetal heart rate. There may be other causes of a non-reactive test, the most common being that the test is conducted when the baby is asleep. For this reason, if the test appears non-reactive, efforts may be made to wake the baby up, which can be done by manipulating the uterus or stimulating the baby. Often, an artificial larynx is placed against the uterus, and turned on to essentially wake the baby up. It's used here as a kind of fetal alarm clock.

A reactive test strongly indicates a healthy baby. Stillbirths within seven days of a reactive non-stress test are rare. For this reason, in most situations where the non-stress test is performed, it's done once or twice a week as long as the test remains reactive.

A non-reactive test on the other hand, may not necessarily mean that the baby is in jeopardy. One of the other tests mentioned below may be recommended to further evaluate the situation.

The Contraction Stress Test

Contractions squeeze the placenta, which will tell the doctor what the oxygen situation is like for the baby. The only time a contraction stress test is done is when the doctor suspects that a fetus may not survive labor as a result of a preexisting health problem of yours, or a fetal development problem. There are three methods of doing this test.

You'll be hooked up to fetal heart monitor and be observed for contractions. If you're having contractions on your own, the contractions are monitored, and the fetal heart is observed for deceleration (any perceived decrease in heart rate after the contraction).

If you're not having contractions on your own, you'll be asked to play with your nipples, which will trigger the hormone oxytocin (discussed more in chapters 8 and 9), the hormone responsible for making your uterus "go." If that fails, you'll be given synthetic oxytocin in small amounts to induce a contraction.

A negative contraction stress test means "everything is normal"; there are no abnormal decelerations of the fetal heart rate. A suspicious contraction stress test may show some deceleration, but not enough to warrant a positive result. Usually, a suspicious test is repeated within 24 hours. In an abnormal or positive test result, there are repeated abnormal decelerations. The treatment will depend on the preexisting condition that warrants the test in the first place. Delivery may be recommended, and in some circumstances, induction of labor may be attempted. In others, delivery by cesarean may be a better idea.

If you have an "unsatisfactory" test result, meaning that you are having too few contractions or the doctor cannot pick up the fetal heart rate, retesting at a later date will be necessary.

Sometimes there are too many contractions to get a good reading on the fetal heartrate. This is known as "hyperstimulation." If you're hyperstimulated, you'll need to retake the test at a later date as well.

Who should not have a contraction stress test?

A contraction stress test isn't for everyone. You may not be able to have a contraction stress test if you:

- have had an episode of premature labor during your pregnancy;
- have an incompetent cervix;
- have already ruptured your membranes;
- are having a multiple pregnancy;
- have polyhydramnios (see chapter 4);
- have a vertical C-section scar (as opposed to a horizontal scar, see chapter 7); or
- have either placenta previa or abruption.

If you do fall into one of these categories, you can certainly have the non-stress test or the biophysical profile, discussed next.

The Biophysical Profile

This test begins with a non-stress test, but then uses ultrasound to check for specific fetal health signs. Each sign of health scores two points, and the overall score makes up what's known as a "biophysical profile" of the fetus. Essentially, the doctor is looking for four basic things on the ultrasound: fetal breathing movements, fetal body movements, fetal muscle tone, and the amount of amniotic fluid.

A score of 4 or less is abnormal; 6 is borderline; 8 or 10 is normal. If you have an abnormal or borderline test, delivering the baby may be considered but this greatly depends on what the problem is, how your own health is and so on. If the baby is still quite premature, and you have an abnormal or borderline score, you may need to retest at a later date.

As your due date approaches, you and your partner are, in a sense, walking off a high-rise window ledge and taking a leap of faith. Every labor and delivery experience, no matter how typical, is challenging. You need to be prepared for any combination of experiences: sudden labor/quick delivery; prolonged and difficult labor/prolonged vaginal delivery; unremarkable labor that turns into a cesarean section because of fetal distress; or reporting, postterm, to your hospital for induction. These are only four of hundreds of combinations of experiences you may have. In the next chapter you'll learn all about labor and delivery: cesareans, delivery of twins, episiotomies, and every imaginable issue regarding this area. So get into position, and get ready to read about the big day!

7

All About
Labor and Delivery

Even in a book devoted to pregnancy, it's difficult to capture the essence of every imaginable labor and delivery experience. What you'll find here is all the information you need to prepare you for a variety of labor and delivery scenarios. This chapter discusses induction, natural labor, and pain relief, as well as problems that necessitate surgical intervention, such as fetal distress. You'll also find a complete section on vaginal and surgical deliveries (forceps, vacuum extraction, and cesarean sections). For most of you, the birth of the placenta will follow delivery of your baby; for some of you, another baby will follow! That's why I've included information on the birth of a second twin. Although premature labor is discussed in chapter 6, whether you experience labor prematurely, right on schedule, or well past your due date, this chapter is designed to meet the information "requirements" of every mother about to deliver.

I've provided a detailed section on "emergency childbirth procedures," using the actual first-aid instructions provided to 911 callers in this situation. I hope none of you will ever need to use these instructions, but it's important that both you and your partner are prepared.

When you're finished reading this, I encourage you to make two copies of these instructions, one for yourself and one for your partner, who should familiarize himself with these procedures, just in case. Keep these instructions with you at all times.

Your "To Do" List

The last two weeks of pregnancy can be filled with anxiety, impatience, and *boredom*. So while you're waiting to be reproductive, you can also be productive by making the appropriate arrangements for your hospital stay and return home with your new baby.

First, if you and your partner have not yet had a tour of your hospital or birthing facility, DO IT TODAY! It's important to see where you will be laboring, delivering, and recovering. (This is discussed more in chapter 1.) The next thing you should take care of is pre-registering at the hospital; you can do this when you take your tour.

You'll then need to have a sort of "dress rehearsal" for the hospital, which may seem like a "Lucy Ricardo" type of practice but a necessary one for most of you. From home, drive yourself to the hospital (or have someone drive you) during rush-hour traffic as well as off-peak hours. Time yourself in both scenarios so you know how much time you'll need to get to the hospital. For example, if your contractions are coming 30 minutes apart, but it takes 2 hours in traffic to get to the hospital, you'll need to leave sooner than a woman who lives around the corner from the hospital!

Another important feature of good planning is making sure your car works. Get it tuned up NOW so you can rely on it when you're in labor. If you don't have a car, make sure you have reliable transportation to get to the hospital. Do not rely on public transportation! Arrange for a friend or family member to be available, or prearrange with a taxi company to come and get you.

The Right Stuff

I hate to sound like your mother, but do you really know what to pack for your "hospital bag"? It's surprising how little thought can go into this rather important piece of luggage. But having the right "stuff" can really transform your labor experience:

- Feel-good toiletries. If you enjoy talcum powder, peppermint foot cream from The Body Shop, or aromatherapeutic oils, bring them! You'll want to be massaged and pampered throughout labor.
- Lip balm. You'll be doing a lot of hard work and a lot of sweating, and you'll feel chapped and dehydrated. You'll need this.
- Juice or bottled water, gum, mints, mouthwash, etc. You'll have a dry throat and dry mouth and may need to be refreshed. (Depending on your situation, you may not be allowed to drink and will be put on an IV. Gum is fine, however.)
- Coach's goodie bag. Your coach is going to get hungry while you're in labor. To avoid "Honey, I'm going upstairs to grab something to eat," while you desperately want him at your side, pack non-perishable food snacks for him.
- Extra pillows. Hospitals never give you enough pillows, and when they do, the pillows always seem to be stuffed with foam core. So bring some from home in colored pillowcases, with your name on them, so the hospital knows they're yours.
- Enough lounge clothes for two days. Whether it's frilly night-gowns or sweatpants and T-shirts, pack two changes of clothes. A bathrobe and slippers/slip-ons are also a good idea. Make sure whatever you bring can accommodate a sore crotch area and possibly a tender abdominal area.
- Necessary toiletries. To avoid saying "You didn't bring my tooth-brush!" pack one now along with a brush, comb, hair dryer, toothpaste, soap, makeup (for your visitors), and deodorant.
- Film and camera equipment. There's no better photo opportunity than birth. Make sure you have film, flashes, video cameras, whatever.

- Woman's stuff. A box of maxi-pads (hospitals do provide these, but you may want to use your own brand) with "wings," two nursing bras, and *cotton* panties. You'll thank me later.
- Your phone book. You'll want to call everyone and their dog once your baby(ies) arrives, so make sure you know where to reach them!
- Baby stuff. Install your infant car seat now. If your baby room is ready, fill it with diapers, plastic pants, sleepers, a receiving blanket, and appropriate baby clothes for the climate. If you're superstitious and don't believe in purchasing any of these things until the baby is born, your partner can do this in a day before you come home.

The Birth Plan

Your practitioner will most likely sit down with you sometime before your due date to discuss your labor and delivery "wish list." In other words, who will be coaching you, what your feelings are about pain relief, what position you'd like to deliver in, and what procedures you absolutely refuse, regardless of the circumstances. For example, if you're carrying a child with Down's syndrome, although you opted not to terminate (discussed in chapter 5), you may still refuse any intervention even if the fetus is in distress. This decision may help you accept what nature truly has in store for you. On the other hand, you may be staunchly against pain relief and want the experience to be as natural as possible. You therefore can make known your objections to epidurals (discussed below) at this point.

You may want to feel as little pain as is medically possible and welcome pain relief and intervention in the hopes of "getting it over with" as quickly as possible. None of these decisions is right or wrong, but they must be the right decisions for you.

It's crucial to note, though, that the birth plan often is just a "wish list." Any number of problems can arise that will warrant more or less intervention than you'd like.

When You're Induced

Having your labor induced is a common experience. Known as induction, this will be done if either your health or the womb's environment sours for some reason (as is the case in many postmature pregnancies) and it's imperative that the baby be delivered. Reasons for induction involve

- Ruptured membranes with a failure to begin labor
- Toxemia (preeclampsia or eclampsia, discussed in chapter 2)
- Chronic or gestational hypertension (see chapter 2)
- Pooped-out placenta, causing postmaturity (see chapter 6)
- Chronic or gestational diabetes—stillbirth is a risk for too long a gestation period, so labor is usually induced by 40 weeks (see chapter 2 for more details)
- Anyone two weeks past her due date. In most cases, doctors don't want to wait for postmaturity (see chapter 6) to set in, so they'll induce you.

Your doctor will tell you to report to your hospital or birthing facility at a specific time. What's good about this scenario is you can take your time and not feel rushed or panicked about getting to the hospital in time. The bad news is that you may experience a more painful labor because it's brought on suddenly, and an epidural may be necessary.

Methods of Induction

There are three methods used to induce labor. No method is right or wrong; it simply depends on what your doctor prefers doing. When you're told you need to be induced, you might want to ask your doctor about the method used and ask for an alternative method if you're not comfortable.

Artificial rupture of membranes (AROM)

If the baby's head has engaged and you experience the lightening discussed in chapter 6, your doctor may decide to "break your water" (the membranes that surround the baby) manually by inserting a device called an amnihook into your vagina. This device looks like a crochet hook. When this is done, either a syntocinon drip or prostaglandin gel may follow (discussed below). Occasionally, no medications are used and your labor usually follows shortly after. If your baby's head has not engaged or its lie is not appropriate (see chapter 6), AROM isn't possible.

These membranes contain amniotic fluid (clear, yellowish fluid that may look like urine), which is the baby's own urine and skin cells. Since the baby floats comfortably on these membranes, when the membranes are broken the baby will start its "descent."

You can expect to feel a gushing of fluid from your vagina when this happens. This is where sanitary pads will come in handy, and your hospital staff may protect the bed with a rubber sheet. When membranes rupture naturally prior to natural labor, this is known as either premature rupture of membranes (PROM), when it's more than 24 hours prior to onset contractions, or spontaneous rupture of membranes (SROM), when it happens shortly before or during labor. PROM is discussed below.

Syntocinon drip

To date, this has been the most widely used method of induction in North America. Syntocinon is just synthetic oxytocin, your body's "labor hormone." Normally, your body produces oxytocin prior to the onset of labor. Oxytocin is what makes your uterus "go," causing it to contract. Nipple stimulation will also trigger oxytocin. This is discussed briefly in chapter 4 and in more detail in chapter 9.

In this case, syntocinon is given to you intravenously. The dosage will vary on how soon your contractions begin and how they progress. The baby's condition will also be monitored as you receive the drip. This drip may be combined with AROM. The intensity and pain associated with your contractions following this method will vary; some women have painful labor, some don't. Your experience will be comparable to natural labor. You'll also experience the stages of labor discussed below.

Prostaglandin gel

Widely used in the United Kingdom and increasingly in North

America, this gel mimics the body's natural prostaglandins, also released during labor, causing the uterus to contract. The gel is applied directly to the cervix and can sometimes assist with dilating the cervix. The benefit is that you're not chained to an IV; however, if you need other fluids such as glucose or salt, the IV is already in place with syntocinon. Prostaglandin gel is believed to induce labor contractions more gently. AROM may accompany this method. Again, you'll then go into the natural stages of labor.

Natural Labor

Labor isn't a swift process. Unlike what sitcoms lead us to believe, most women have time to get to the hospital, even if they go into a "sudden labor." If you need to be induced, you'll experience all the phases of labor in the hospital and will report to the hospital feeling fine. Labor is divided into three segments: pre-labor, early labor, and active labor. Then, you "graduate" to delivery, discussed separately.

Pre-labor

Pre-labor can begin anywhere in the last few weeks or last days of pregnancy. And, of course, many women will experience this prematurely and past their due date. This is when you experience lightening, and begin to feel more pressure on your bladder. You may get diarrhea and possibly a severe backache, both precursors to early labor. The diarrhea is "nature's enema" and is your body's way of emptying everything out before actual labor begins. You'll also feel the Braxton Hicks contractions more frequently (these are painless).

Your cervix softens at this stage and may start to thin out and dilate slightly. The mucus plug that seals the cervical opening starts to break, causing a mucusy, bloody discharge, which is charmingly referred to as "bloody show" or "show." You may even expel the entire plug—which will look like a glob of pink jelly with some blood on it.

Premature rupture of membranes (PROM)

Membranes more commonly rupture after contractions have set in, not before. If more than 24 hours pass before onset contractions, this is officially premature rupture of membranes (PROM). As the baby's head presses down on the amniotic membranes that contain fluid, the membranes may break. This is what's known as breaking your water, the classic pre-labor symptom. Women expect this event to be like a flood of water suddenly rushing out of their vaginas. It frequently happens this way, but the fluid may also just trickle out. It will be clear, odorless, and milky. Some women think they've wet their pants when this happens. Sometimes your water doesn't break and it happens during more active labor. If it doesn't, don't worry about it.

Now is a good time to get ready to go to the hospital! Some women may choose to stay home until active labor begins (see below). This is an individual decision and depends on how "high risk" your pregnancy is, how anxious you are, and a hundred other things you'll have been prepared for by your practitioner. For the purposes of this chapter, I'll assume that all phases of labor take place in the hospital. If your water has broken, you'll need to follow some special commonsense hygiene practices. Showers instead of baths is an obvious one. Your practitioner and midwife will give you more instructions as well. Your doctor or midwife (or whoever is on staff at the hospital) will also want to examine you vaginally to see how much your cervix is dilating. The "real stuff" of labor—the more active phases—begins anytime between 1 and 24 hours after your water breaks. If the membranes have been ruptured for 24 hours or more, and you're not in labor, induction will probably be considered, discussed earlier in the chapter. If it doesn't break, the bloody show is also a sign that labor is beginning, and your doctor may choose to perform AROM.

Early Labor

Pre-labor slowly unfolds into early labor. This phase lasts about seven or eight hours. You may not even notice a change in the process, however. Early labor and active labor are also known as the first stage of labor, the effacement and dilation stage. Early labor is characterized by contractions that cause the cervix to dilate about 3–4 centimeters. These contractions can feel sort of wave-like. They build up, then recede. They will be mildly painful and begin in the lower back. They can also feel like heavy menstrual cramps. At this point you may want to start practicing what you learned in your childbirth classes in terms of breathing, relaxing, and so on. At this point, the contractions will be anywhere from 5 to 20 minutes apart, become more intense each time they occur, last anywhere from 30–45 seconds, get longer each time they occur, and get closer together. (If you're not in the hospital already, you'll need to go in for sure when the contractions are about 5 minutes apart. The contractions may also become more pronounced with walking.) You'll be able to sleep, eat, and engage in normal activities throughout this phase.

Active labor

Active labor is similar to early labor but is far more pronounced. This phase lasts 3–5 hours or longer. If you're sleeping, for example, you'll be woken up by the intensity of these contractions. Now the contractions occur every 2–4 minutes and last up to 60 seconds. They may be moderately painful or extremely painful, depending on the woman. At this phase, keep emptying your bladder regularly. If you're offered an epidural, a painkiller that numbs you from the breasts down (discussed below) do it now. You will have a choice and the right to accept or refuse it. An epidural will take the edge off your pain, but you may want to feel everything. With an epidural you'll also need to remain in bed because your legs will now be numb. At this point, the cervix will continue to dilate. When it's fully dilated, it measures about 10 centimeters. Active labor encompasses the transition phase (anywhere from 8–10 centimeters), which is discussed further below. Epidural or not, you may also get an incredible urge to push, which mirrors the urge to push out a bowel movement. You may also start to feel either very warm or chilly. At this stage, your nurse, midwife, or practitioner will continuously check your cervical dilation via vaginal examination, and your baby's heartbeat. With an epidural, an intravenous line will be started as well as an electronic fetal heart monitor, if they haven't already. You'll also need to use a bedpan if you've had the epidural.

A Word About Pain Management

Don't let anyone tell you that labor isn't painful; it is. But your perception of pain and your threshold for pain will determine whether a painkiller is "indicated" or not.

Getting pain relief during childbirth does not in any way mean that you are "medicalizing" your childbirth experience; it means that you are humanizing the experience. Natural childbirth is an overused, rather passé term that does little to help women make an informed decision about pain management. Believe me, if the medicinal benefits of the 1990s were available in the 1890s, few women would have refused them. So bear in mind, while you're bearing down, that the Natural Childbirth Movement was a necessary outgrowth of a male-dominated obstetrics industry that was insensitive to maternity patients' needs. Today, the obstetrics industry is at least 50% female and geared toward the best interests of the mother and child. Pain relief is an option designed to make you more comfortable, not more dependent or powerless. It's also important to note that painkillers may not completely free you of discomfort or pain.

Finally, you have a choice regarding pain relief, and you can make your preferences known to your practitioners when you discuss your birth plan. There are a variety of painkillers that can be used, including pudendal blocks, caudal anesthesia, epidural anesthesia (the most popular choice), paracervical block anesthesia, and narcotics such as pethidine, morphine, or others. There are also non-medicinal routes such as breathing techniques, hypnosis, and acupuncture. Discuss with your practitioner all of the pain relief options as well as the anticipated difficulty of delivery (your baby's positioning, your bone structure, and so on). Then, plan for a few different labor experiences in either the easier or more difficult direction. If the labor is easier than expected, forego the pain relief; if it's more difficult, you'll have the pain relief there when you want it.

The epidural

An epidural is not just reserved for childbirth; it's used in a variety of gynecological and orthopedic procedures. By far the most popular and widely available pain relief method, an epidural offers tremendous pain relief during labor. It can also serve as an anesthesia during complicated labor and delivery and delivery by cesarean section. It's also safer than narcotics or general anesthesia, which is why it's so popular.

Before the epidural is administered, an intravenous will be set up so various fluids can be dripped into you if necessary, preventing falling blood volume, low blood pressure, and so on. You'll be asked to either curl up into a ball with your back facing the anesthesiologist, or to sit on the edge of the bed with your back facing him or her. Your back will be swabbed with antiseptic. Then, a needle is injected into the space between the spinal cord and the bones of your back. You'll be asked to keep very still since the needle is close to the spinal cord. When the needle is in position, a tube is threaded through the inside of the needle. The needle is removed, the tube is taped to your back, and the anesthetic is injected into the tube. In about 20 minutes, your nerves in that area are numbed, and you may need either a bed pan or bladder catheter since your bladder is also numbed. The epidural wears off around the time you deliver.

Of all women on epidurals, 90% find acceptable pain relief from it, and 50% find complete pain relief. If the tube bends or too little anesthetic is administered, pain relief may not be as complete as it should be.

What are the drawbacks?

Some practitioners feel that epidurals may interfere with pushing, prolonging delivery or causing more intervention via forceps or vacuum extraction. In addition, while some studies conclude that epidurals are associated with longer labors, it must also be noted that it is primarily longer labors where epidurals are most needed. If the epidural is done in very early labor, it could increase the risk of a cesarean section. More-over, there has been anecdotal evidence suggesting that epidurals may lead to future chronic back pain, but this hasn't been clinically proven. Finally, an epidural can be administered only by a skilled anesthesiologist or obstetrician in a hospital setting, and cannot be given to women who are dehydrated, hemorrhaging, or have low blood pressure. Epidurals may be fine for women with high blood pressure, but it depends on the situation.

Transition Phase

This phase takes you into delivery and lasts anywhere from 30 to 90 minutes. If you haven't had any pain medication, the scenario is that you've been in active labor for approximately three hours now. You may be tired, abusive, and frustrated, and have no clue what time it is. You also may be shaking, hiccuping, vomiting, having chills, cold feet, dry mouth and lips, hyperventilating, moaning, crying, or screaming. Mean-while, you feel rectal pressure and have a *TREMENDOUS* urge to push. Your contractions are the most intense now, occurring every 30 seconds and lasting 90 seconds, and your cervix is almost fully dilated. Some women may want to go to the toilet, which will help them relax and get the pushing going. If you've had an epidural, the transition phase may come and go without your feeling any significant change in your physique. Often, women with an epidural may just sit quietly chatting with their partner or coach, or may even just watch television. You may still experience shaking because of the epidural, and you may have some nausea, but that's about it. This rather tranquil transition phase may be the best argument for having an epidural.

Delivery: Bearing Down

This is known as the second stage of labor: the descent and delivery portion of labor. Now you can push. Essentially, instead of holding back the urge to push, you'll actually get to do it. This is tough work; your face may turn red and you may be soaked with perspiration. You should push only when you feel the urge to push, however. Try not to force it. The uterus will contract on its own and help the baby out anyway, so waiting for the urge will make the delivery easier for you. In fact, you might be so overwhelmed by the urge to push that you might be frightened by it and hold back.

What does pushing feel like? Pushing during childbirth has often been compared to pushing out a bowel movement. One analogy I came across likened the pushing to, believe it or not, having an orgasm. In other words, no woman can truly describe either one, yet every woman knows how to instinctively have a bowel movement, and most can instinctively climax; it's something that the body just "knows how to do." The only advice one can give regarding having a good orgasm is letting go and allowing yourself to release your sexual energy. Well, it's the same when it comes to pushing; you need to let go and allow your body to take over, to do what it was engineered to do and release its reproductive energy. Bear in mind that if you've had an epidural, the urge to push may be suppressed.

Whatever delivery position you've chosen, you'll be in it by now. Sometimes the position you initially chose will not be the most comfortable, and you may wish to switch. Your pushing may also "push out" some stool (*everyone* does this: don't be embarrassed). In a normal delivery, at this phase, the hardest part is pushing out the head. As the head emerges, you may feel intense burning and stinging sensations, feeling as though you are about to rip apart. If you've had an epidural or a pudendal block (a form of local anesthetic), you won't feel much pain when the head emerges. Most women won't rip apart. The vagina is like a huge elastic band that stretches for this. In fact, some of you may be coerced at this point to consent to an episiotomy (discussed below), but this isn't necessary for uncomplicated deliveries. After you read the episiotomy section, you may want to resist that urge in particular.

The Afterbirth: Birth of the Placenta

This is known as the afterbirth, birth of placenta, or just the third stage of labor. In a vaginal delivery, episiotomy or not, after the birth of the baby your uterus will contract enough to loosen the placenta from the uterine wall. These contractions may be painful but mild in comparison to what you just went through. Besides, you'll be so busy with your newborn that you probably won't even notice them. The placenta will then slip out with one or two pushes. The uterus then continues to contract against exposed blood vessels from where the placenta used to be as a natural way to control bleeding.

Twin Delivery

Each twin will be handled as a single baby, and delivery of one may be easier than the delivery of the second. In approximately 50% of twin births, both babies are in the correct position for a vaginal birth—head down, feet up toward heaven, in a longitudinal (vertical) lie. (See chapter 6 for more details.) As long as all is going well, the babies should be delivered one at a time. The upside in a twin head-first, vaginal delivery is that the heads are usually smaller than a normal single baby and the mother's vagina doesn't need to make as great a stretch to accommodate each head.

In about 40% of all twin deliveries, one twin is in the correct position, while the other twin is in a breech position (feet, knees, or buttocks first). Vaginal deliveries may still be possible as long as a skilled obstetrician is handling the birth. Squatting positions may also be used to help the breech delivery. In addition, since the heads in twin birth are smaller, the complication involved with a stuck head is not as great in a twin breech delivery as it is in a single breech delivery.

Nevertheless, because of the challenge of a twin delivery, most mothers of twins can expect to have some kind of intervention. How much intervention you have depends on the doctor's skill. It also depends on which twin is breech. For example, if the first twin is breech and the second is in the correct position, virtually no doctor will allow a vaginal delivery; you'll need a cesarean section. If, however, the first twin is headfirst, and the second twin is breech, you may be able to deliver both vaginally. Occasionally, a cesarean section may be necessary to deliver that second twin. The afterbirth will then involve either one large placenta or two placentas.

When Something Goes Wrong

This time, when something goes wrong, it usually has to do with the baby's presentation or "lie" not being compatible with a vaginal delivery (if it's breech or in a horizontal position—discussed in chapter 6), or a structural problem with you that does not allow a natural vaginal delivery to take place. For example, if your cervix isn't dilating enough, this is a problem; if your vaginal opening is too small for the baby's head, this is a problem; and if the fetus goes into distress, this is an emergency!

Fetal Distress

Fetal distress is a vague term that refers to several problems that can result in a stillbirth (discussed further in chapter 6). Once your membranes rupture, the baby must be born within a reasonable time. It cannot stay inside because there's no more cushioning for it, and bacteria can enter its environment, causing infections. Fetal distress can occur when there isn't enough oxygen through the placenta or there is pressure on the umbilical cord. Fetal distress is usually diagnosed by changes in the fetal heart rate pattern. If this is suspected, your doctor may try to change your position, give you oxygen or give you more intravenous fluids, which may improve the baby's condition, and allow labor to continue. However, if the baby doesn't respond within a short while, the baby will need to be delivered by the quickest route possible.

The bottom line is this: As soon as you hear the words "the baby (or fetus) is in distress," alarm bells should go off in your head. Forget the birth plan and prepare for the quickest delivery route. The baby needs to get out—NOW! Whether this means delivery via episiotomy, cesarean, forceps, or vacuum extraction (all discussed below), your doctor will need to intervene and get your baby out of its hostile environment ASAP.

The Episiotomy

An episiotomy is a minor surgical procedure where an incision is made into the perineum, the area between your rectum and vagina. It's done to enlarge the opening for vaginal births, making it easier for the baby's head to come out. You will probably be given a local anesthetic for this between contractions, but if you've had an epidural, you won't need it. After the birth, the area is frozen via local anesthetic, and you'll be sewn back together.

On the general consent form you sign when you register as a maternity patient, there is usually a space for your signature consenting to this procedure. Before you sign it, you should discuss alternatives to episiotomies with your practitioner or midwife, and find out when the procedure is truly necessary. Some women find this an uncomfortable procedure and a hindrance to the overall childbirth experience. In addition, the procedure is necessary only about 25% of the time, even though it's almost always performed.

Why is that? All doctors will tell you that they perform an episiotomy only when it's necessary. This is not so. First, the doctor that tells you this, as discussed in chapter 1, may not be delivering you. Meanwhile, the resident or intern who's on call in OB-Gyn when you go into labor may do an episiotomy for any number of reasons; usually, these reasons have to do with a mistrust of natural vaginal engineering.

Most vaginas have an incredible Lycra quality to them. But doctors usually don't wait around to witness the Lycra vagina; they just make the cut, which they consider minor. The routine episiotomy cuts through skin, vaginal mucosa, and three layers of muscle in an otherwise sensitive area. The side effects include pain, bleeding, a breakdown of stitches, and delayed healing. The pain afterward can be enough to keep you from you sitting comfortably for several weeks—the last thing you need when you're nursing a newborn. One of the few studies that have been done on the side effects of this procedure show that 6 percent of women who had episiotomies suffer from persistent pain during sexual intercourse following the procedure.

Remember, midwives are trained to deliver babies without the assistance of surgery. That's why a good midwife, combined with a good hospital, is the best system. The midwife will "watch over you" during delivery and can help gauge whether your vagina can make the stretch it was designed to make. Midwives can also do episiotomies if necessary. Many doctors believe that a little natural tearing, which will often take place without the episiotomy, will not only heal much quicker than a surgical tearing, but is less painful.

When is an episiotomy necessary?

Any medical emergency during delivery. Some examples: when the baby is in distress (as discussed above); to facilitate the delivery of a premature or breech baby; whenever forceps are necessary (necessary when the head is an awkward position).

The procedure is also necessary when the delivery of the baby's head is progressing at a rate or manner that will badly tear the perineum, or in some cases, when the vagina isn't making the stretch. Other legitimate reasons for an episiotomy include:

- the prevention of damaging tears in the rectal area, causing potential prolapse or incontinence in the future;
- preventing old pregnancy tears from opening (from past perineum tears); or
- shortening labor for women suffering from heart conditions,

hypertension, or clear mental and physical exhaustion (when you're exhausted, the risk of fetal distress is higher).

For the majority of normal, vaginal deliveries, the episiotomy is not necessary.

Forceps Delivery

Has your toast ever gotten stuck in the toaster? Of course! What do you use to get it out? Tongs. Well, that's exactly what a forceps delivery is, except the "toaster" is your vagina, the "toast" is your baby, and the forceps are the "tongs." In fact, forceps were once upon a time a trade secret of one particular doctor who looked after an important family. This family had an unusually high rate of healthy childbirths as a result.

Forceps are truly necessary when delivery of the head is a struggle and delays birth for an unreasonable amount of time. For a variety of reasons, the labor can progress, delivery is imminent, and then, something, quite literally, gets stuck. Has the baby turned? Is your pelvis too small? Can you not seem to make the last push? It really doesn't matter what the reasons are. The point behind the forceps delivery is to "clear" the head of your vagina ASAP. Most forceps deliveries are incredibly fast, lasting 2–10 minutes. First, you'll have an episiotomy. Then the forceps are inserted and ever so gently, applied to either side of the baby's head, drawing it out. Now, imagine trying to dig out your toast without breaking it. Well, the same principles of physics apply here; gentle maneuvering is the key to a forceps delivery. And, with a skilled obstetrician, they are almost always non-traumatic, quick, and successful to the point that you may not even be aware it is happening. It's important to distinguish between the forceps deliveries of 30 years ago and those done today. In 1995, only "easy" forceps deliveries are done, in the sense that there is no risk of damaging the baby's head due to intense tugging or pulling. If there is any perceived risk to the baby at all, a cesarean section will be done. In 1965, however, cesarean sections weren't as commonly done, and more risky forceps deliveries were attempted.

Vacuum Extraction

Has your drain ever been clogged? Of course! What do you use to un-clog it? A plunger. This is what happens in a vacuum extraction, except your vagina is the "drain," your baby is the "clog," and the "plunger" is the vacuum.

Just as in a forceps scenario, something gets stuck that requires in-tervention. A small suction cup, designed like a miniature plunger, is in-serted into the vagina, and attached to the baby's head. A small hand pump creates the suction action and pulls out the head.

Now, you could probably use tongs to get at the clog and dig, but a plunger is more efficient and will do a better job. Similarly, vacuum extraction in some circumstances is a more efficient way to unclog a stopped head. Vacuum extraction is necessary for the same reasons for-ceps may be necessary, but are usually reserved for heads that are stuck higher up the pelvis, rather than lower. The good news about vacuum extractions is that an episiotomy may not be necessary. And there's less risk of injury to the vaginal tissues. Because of this, vacuum extractions are growing in popularity. One side effect is a minor swelling called a "chignon" on the baby's head as a result of the cup. This is nothing to be alarmed about; it will go away. Scalp injuries from the newer vacuum extraction methods are uncommon. You'd have the same thing if some-one suctioned your head.

The Cesarean Birth

About one in four babies is delivered by cesarean section. A cesarean section, or C-section, is a surgical procedure that is essentially "abdomi-nal delivery." The procedure, as the name suggests, dates back to Julius Caesar, who, as legend tells us, was born in this manner. Whether Cae-sar truly was a cesarean birth is hotly debated among historians, but what historians do know is that the abdominal delivery dates back to ancient Rome. In fact, Roman law made it legal to perform a cesarean section only if the mother died in the last four weeks of pregnancy. The procedure therefore originated only as a means to save the child. Using the procedure to save the mother was not even considered until the 19th century, under the influence of two prominent obstetricians, Max Sanger and Eduardo Porro.

This is considered major pelvic surgery that usually involves either a spinal or epidural (only in some cases is a general anesthetic necessary). A vertical or horizontal incision is made just above your pubic hair line (you may need to be shaved for this). Then the surgeon (usually) cuts horizontally through the uterine muscle and eases the baby out. Sometimes this second cut is vertical, known as the classic incision. It is this second cut, into the uterine muscle, that will allow a VBAC (Vaginal Birth After Cesarean) or not. With a horizontal cut, women have gone on to have normal second vaginal births; with the classic cut, the scar is less stable and will mean that for you, "once a C-section, always a C-section" is a reality.

In some instances, you'll know in advance whether you need to have a cesarean section. Your pelvis may be too small; you may have irreparable scarring on your cervix from previous pelvic surgery that will prevent dilation, or an emergency situation may be detected that requires the fetus to be taken out immediately.

A Dozen Good Reasons to Have a C-Section

Below are 12 legitimate reasons why a cesarean section may be performed.

1. A prolonged labor, caused by failure to dilate, failure of the labor to progress, too large a head, and several other reasons.
2. A failed induction attempt. (Induction sometimes fails, and when the baby is overdue, a cesarean is the next alternative. See above for more details on induction.)
3. When the baby is in a breech position. (See chapter 6 for more details, as well the twin delivery section above.)

4. Placental problems (see chapter 6 for more details).
5. Fetal distress (see above).
6. Health problems, such as toxemia or hypertension.
7. A history of difficult deliveries or stillbirth.
8. When the baby is in a transverse lie (horizontal position), discussed in chapter 6.
9. When a vaginal delivery, even with intervention, is risky.
10. When the mother has active genital herpes (see chapters 1 and 2).
11. Structural problems such as fibroids or other pelvic abnormalities that prevent normal vaginal delivery.
12. Some multiple births (see also twin delivery section above).

Unnecessary vs. Necessary Cesareans

Many unnecessary cesarean sections are performed. If the uterine cut was horizontal, most second cesareans are not necessary. Another common practice is to perform a C-section when a woman fails to go into labor after being induced. Reasons for being induced usually have to do with progressing past the due date. You may wish to get a second opinion about your induction before you go ahead. In a U.S. study, situations where a C-section was performed depended more on the doctor than on any other single factor; the rate of C-sections varied from 19% to 42%, according to the individual doctor's preference. This is a huge discrepancy. What it boils down to is the doctor's definition of "emergency," which may arise in the event of any of the problems listed above. No competent doctor will delay a C-section if he or she thinks the labor is endangering the baby's or mother's health.

To avoid an unnecessary procedure, consult with your practitioner and midwife *before* the third trimester. Find out what situations truly warrant a C-section and whether you're a VBAC candidate. If you're experiencing a difficult or high-risk pregnancy (see chapter 2) or will be having a multiple birth you may be more likely to have the procedure than a woman with a low-risk pregnancy.

Knowing the "Score"

After the baby is delivered, its breathing is attended to, and it is weighed and measured. As if all this laboring and delivering weren't enough, the last hurdle is knowing your baby's health "score." I'm not making this up—your baby is given one point for every health hurdle she or he passes immediately after birth. Seven and above is a good score, 10 is a perfect score. Five signs of health are judged according to the Apgar score:

- breathing (a weak cry and slow breathing score 1 point; a strong cry scores 2 points)
- pulse (under 100 beats per minute scores 1 point; over 100 beats scores 2 points)
- color (good body color with blue fingers or toes scores 1 point; all-over pink scores 2)
- muscular tone (flexing of fingers or toes scores 1; active flexing and kicking scores 2)
- response to annoying gestures—called *response to stimuli* (grimaces score 1 point; crying scores 2)

If your baby scores 0 (not breathing; no pulse; blue and pale; limp; not responding to stimuli), or under 7, he or she will need immediate neonatal care. Testing may begin in another 5 minutes after a problem is examined.

Childbirth 911: Emergency Childbirth Procedures

Emergency childbirth procedures are necessary when you go into labor (either at term or prematurely) and you have no time or no way of getting to a hospital or birthing facility. The sole intention of anyone's practicing first aid in this instance is to assist you in delivering the baby and to protect you and the baby until you can be transported to a hospital or appropriate facility for further care. The following instructions are intended to be used in emergency situations only, and must coincide with a 911 call for an ambulance, if possible. They are not intended as instructions for a pre-planned home birth delivery.

As I stated earlier, two sets of these instructions should be copied; one set needs to stay with you at all times (in your wallet or purse), while the other set should remain with your partner. Whether you're in a taxi cab, stuck in hopeless traffic, at work, traveling abroad, or on your kitchen floor about to deliver, these instructions should go to the first available person, who must help you deliver the child. This is why the instructions are written in simple language. Whether this person is your coworker, neighbor, housekeeper, spouse, mother, or taxi driver, these instructions should be passed on to him or her immediately while he or she calls 911 and requests an ambulance.

Ready-to-Deliver Instructions

Whoever you are, these instructions will help you safely deliver this woman's baby. Your first priority is assisting this woman and protecting her and her baby until the ambulance can get there. If you're near a phone, before you begin assisting, please call 911 or instruct someone else to do so. Make sure you give the address or identifiable landmarks (i.e., "corner of Smith and Jones, in a red car across from the church") to the 911 operator so the ambulance can get there ASAP. If your 911 operator gives you alternate instructions or tells you to stand by, follow that advice. If things progress and delivery seems unavoidable, or if you have no way of getting to a phone, take a deep breath and read on.

You will be delivering three things: a **baby** (called a fetus when it is still unborn), a **placenta** (a large, flat, spongy organ that is attached to the wall of the woman's **uterus** (the lower part of her stomach area, where the fetus develops), and an **umbilical cord,** a cord-like organ that attaches to the baby's belly button and the placenta. The placenta and the umbilical cord nourish and feed the baby. ***Under no circum-stances should you attempt to cut the umbilical cord.*** The baby, the um-bilical cord, and the placenta will be delivered from the **cervix,** an opening that leads to the uterus (called the neck of the uterus), which will probably be dilated. The woman's **vagina** leads to her cervix. The baby will be coming out of the vagina (also called a birth canal).

Is there time to get to a hospital?

If this woman is having **contractions,** which means the baby is moving down her uterus, toward her vagina, she will be in pain. Re-move her panties if this is not already done and check the opening of her vagina for any fluid, blood, or mucous. Contractions, accompanied by fluid, blood, and/or mucous mean only that the first stage of labor has begun. In this case, there should be enough time to get to the hospi-tal. If the contractions become stronger, last longer, and are more fre-quent, there may not be time to get to the hospital. If she needs to move her bowels, or if you can see the baby's head through the opening of the vagina, the second stage of labor has begun and you will need to assist in delivering the baby.

What You Need to Do Now: Preparation for Delivery

1. Find a helper, preferably a woman.
2. Wash your hands thoroughly and gather the following materials:
   - clean towels to drape over the woman and dry off the new-born at birth (the newborn will be wet and slippery). Clean sheets (flannel is best) can also be used.
   - a soft blanket to wrap up the newborn after it's delivered.
   - a plastic bag with ties to hold the placenta and the umbilical cord (you'll need to save these).
   - soap, water, and towels to wash your hands throughout this process.

- sterile, narrow roller bandage or tape in case you need to tie off the umbilical cord (explained later).
- sanitary napkins to soak up uterine bleeding.

Check to see if she has any of these items with her in a packed "hospital bag." If you are at her home, check the washroom and baby's room for some of these things, too.

3. Ask her to lie or sit down in the most comfortable position she can. Encourage her to lie down on her back with her knees bent. This will make the delivery easier for you. Support her back with pillows or "substitute" pillows like a rolled-up coat or towel.

4. Once she is comfortable, cover her with sheets and towels so she can maintain some privacy and dignity. This will help to calm her down. You should also reassure this woman and try to act calm and unhurried.

5. Place clean towels or a sheet under this woman's buttocks (rear end), extending them between her thighs. Place a clean towel between her legs so you can lay the newborn on it after birth.

The "Head First" Delivery (normal delivery)

Remember, do not attempt to interfere with the natural course of events. You should be assisting only, ensuring that the newborn is safely delivered out from the vagina and protected until help arrives.

The baby's head will come out of the vagina first and should turn to one side to allow the shoulders to pass through the vaginal opening. Try to prevent the baby's head from emerging too quickly; this could cause injury to the baby. To do this, ask the woman to "hold back" or instruct her "not to push." You can even loudly command "DON'T PUSH" if you need to. The woman will understand what you mean. Meanwhile, GENTLY restrain the baby's head with your hand by putting both hands at either the vaginal opening or on the head itself (if it's partially out) in the STOP position. One hand should cover the rear of the head; the other, the crown-forehead area.

The baby will be covered with a slippery substance called **vernix.**

This makes handling the baby a very slippery business, so be careful. As the baby slips out, gently support the head and the body. If the cord is around the baby's neck, just slowly ease it away by passing it over the head or shoulders. Do not pull or exert any pressure or force on the cord. It should be loose enough for you to just clear it out of the way. If you can, record or note the time of birth.

The "Bottom First" Delivery (breech delivery)

If the baby's buttocks, knees, or feet are coming out first, this is called a **breech delivery.** This is a potentially dangerous situation. Under these circumstances, make every effort to get an ambulance ASAP. In the meantime, support the parts of the baby's body that are coming out of the vagina. Again, the baby will be covered with **vernix.** Try to get the woman to push out the baby's extremities, its abdomen and chest. Once you see the chest area, put both hands under the body and gently lift up and rotate the body back toward the mother's abdomen. This action should enable the baby's mouth and nose to clear the vagina. Clear the airway (see below). The head should follow safely. If the umbilical cord is wrapped around the baby's neck, try to ease it over the head or allow it to slip over the baby's shoulders.

If you can't get the head out safely (if it's stuck and isn't coming out with pushing), keep the parts that are out warm with blankets until help arrives. An expert will help you safely deliver the head.

How to Clear the Baby's Airway

The baby will have fluid in its nose and mouth. This is perfectly normal, but you'll need to clear this fluid away so the baby can begin breathing oxygen.

1. If the baby is entirely out of the vagina, wipe the baby's face with a clean cloth or tissue. You can also try positioning the baby so the lower body and feet are slightly elevated.

2. Because the baby is slippery, use both hands to hold it firmly but gently, keeping it level with the mother's vagina. Use your left hand to hold the baby's feet, with your index finger between the ankles, your thumb around one ankle, and your remaining fingers around the other. Support the back of the baby's head, neck, and shoulders with the other hand.

3. Lift the baby's legs and back slightly, just enough to allow the fluid to drain from the nose and mouth.

4. The baby should be crying as soon as you do this; the face should be turning pink, which means that the baby's lungs are expanding and the baby is breathing. If this isn't happening and the baby is pale and limp, you'll need to perform **artificial respiration:**

   • Open the baby's mouth and lift up the chin. Don't force the head back too far.

   • Don't close the mouth or push on the soft underparts of the chin. This may obstruct the baby's airway.

   • Make a tight seal with your mouth over both the mouth and nose of the baby.

   • Give puffs of air rather than full breaths.

   • If you find a pulse, continue giving artificial respiration and checking the pulse. If you don't find a pulse, don't attempt CPR unless you're trained. Wait for help and keep trying artificial respiration.

5. Once the baby is breathing on its own, make sure that its airway is completely clear. Prevent things like the blankets and towels from obstructing its air passage.

6. The baby must be kept warm. Dry the baby with a clean, warm towel and wrap it in another clean, warm towel or a reasonable substitute. Lay the baby on its side across the mother's abdomen, facing away from the mother's face with its head down. This will help drain excess fluid and make it easier to monitor the baby's breathing.

What to Do with the Umbilical Cord and Placenta

The umbilical cord attached to the baby is also attached to the placenta. The cord is a very delicate organ with veins and arteries. The placenta should come out of the mother's vagina in about 20 minutes or so. To speed things up, you can massage her abdomen. Don't panic if the placenta seems to take a long time to come out. This is normal. **Whatever you do, don't attempt to force out the placenta by pulling on the umbilical cord!**

Once the placenta comes out, make sure it's delivered onto a clean towel. Put it into a clean plastic bag. Make sure that all parts of the placenta and membranes are saved; these need to go to the hospital or medical facility with the mother and baby when help arrives. ***DO NOT UNDER ANY CIRCUMSTANCES ATTEMPT TO CUT THE UMBILICAL CORD!*** Keep the placenta at the same level as the newborn. You can keep it warm inside the newborn's blanket if you like.

If the placenta or cord is bleeding . . .

This shouldn't be happening, but if it does, tie the umbilical cord with clean tape or heavy, thick string at the stem on the baby's abdomen. Do *not* use ordinary string or thread because this may cut the umbilical cord.

Taking Care of the Mother

Once the placenta comes out of the vagina, there will be some bleeding. This is normal. To control the bleeding, you can put your hand on top of the woman's lower abdomen/uterus area and massage it. It will feel like a hard, round mass. Examine the skin between the mother's vagina and anus to see if there are any cuts or tears. If there are, apply pressure to these tears with your fingers. Then get some sanitary napkins to the area to absorb the bleeding. If she is still bleeding heavily, elevate her feet and legs and try to get her to an emergency unit of a hospital ASAP.

The best way to transport the mother and newborn is with the mother lying on her back and the baby securely wrapped in her arms.

Encourage the mother to suckle her newborn on her breast. This will help tighten up her uterus and will control bleeding. It will also help nourish the baby with immunizing antibodies that will help protect the baby from infections.

If the vaginal bleeding doesn't stop . . .

Keep massaging the mother's abdomen and place her in the "shock" position (on her back, head low, and lower extremities raised 6–12 inches to increase the blood flow to the brain). Keep the mother and baby warm and make every effort to get both of them to a medical facility ASAP.

If you've been waiting more than 12 hours for help to arrive . . .

If the mother and baby seem to be well, you can tie or cut the umbilical cord at this point. Here's how you do it:

1. Check the cord for a pulse. If there is a pulse, don't cut it yet; wait for the pulse to stop.
2. After the pulse has stopped, tie or clamp the cord in two places about 3 inches (7 centimeters) apart, positioned about 6–12 inches away from the baby's body.
3. Cut the cord between the two clamps with a pair of sterilized scissors or a sterilized knife.
4. Check the end of the cord and try to control or stop any bleeding.

Again, I hope no one will need to use the above instructions, but being prepared for any circumstance is actually a large part of preparing for labor in general.

All of the issues regarding neonatal care and testing, are covered in a baby and child care book, which this book is not. However, there are a variety of postpartum issues you need to aware of, which are covered in the next three chapters. These issues have to do with your health after childbirth (including your next menstrual period), breastfeeding, and postpartum blues (very important). Enjoy your newborn! Now you can make all your phone calls!

8

Health After Childbirth

If you've had a vaginal delivery, the main reason you need to take extra care after childbirth is because your cervix has been completely dilated. This makes you vulnerable to bacterial infections, which could cause a range of long-term, debilitating gynecological problems. If you've had an episiotomy, you'll need to follow additional hygiene instructions in order for your incision to heal. And if you've had a cesarean section, there are separate after-care issues you'll need to address that have more do to with recovering from major surgery than recovering from childbirth in general.

There are also numerous changes in your body that will start to take place and which require your immediate attention. This chapter will cover all your postpartum discomforts, including the special concerns associated with a high-risk pregnancy. Postpartum exercises, postpartum sex and contraception, and postpartum bleeding are also discussed in detail. Finally, this chapter discusses health problems that can result directly from childbirth. Essentially, everything you need to know about postpartum physical health is here. Breast changes, breastfeeding and breast problems are discussed in chapter 9; postpartum depression is addressed in chapter 10.

The Incredible Shrinking Woman

At the time of delivery, your uterus can weigh as much as 1100 grams, with a volume of 5–10 liters. That's a lot of uterus. Incredibly, after delivery, it immediately begins the process of shrinking in size to its usual 70 grams in weight and 10 milliliters in volume. Your blood volume is also rapidly dropping and will decrease about 45%, causing your heart rate to drop by about 10–15 beats per minute. Your urinary tract is also shrinking. To accommodate the pregnancy, your urinary tract was altered as a result of an increase in blood flow to the area. This changed your kidney function, which is why protein in your urine was such a concern throughout the pregnancy.

As if all these changes weren't enough, you also need to beware of bacteria! As a rule, whenever your cervix is dilated for any reason, be it childbirth, miscarriage, abortion, D & C, therapeutic abortion, cesarean section, or other pelvic surgical procedures, your risk of developing a gynecological infection is at an all-time high. You'll need to avoid getting anything into your vagina for about six weeks or until your cervix has closed up again. This means:

- no swimming—not only can bacteria get into your cervix during swimming, but the chlorine in pools may irritate any tears or incisions.
- no tampons— tampons can act as breeding grounds for bacteria, which then hitchhike up the tampon, entering your cervix.
- no intercourse or sex toys (see the postpartum sex section below).
- no douching—this may alter the vaginal environment and make it less protective against harmful bacteria, while douching might flush vaginal and cervical bacteria into the upper pelvic region.

See your doctor to make sure that the cervix has resumed its usual shape and appearance before you undertake any of the above activities. Also, review basic vaginal hygiene habits discussed under yeast infections in chapter 3. These hygiene rules can also help prevent bacteria from entering your cervix. When bacterial infections do occur, you can develop a condition known as pelvic inflammatory disease (PID), discussed at the end of this chapter.

Your Postpartum ABCs

Again, here's the alphabetical breakdown of postpartum changes and discomforts. After-care for episiotomies and cesarean sections are discussed in separate sections below.

Afterpains (cramps after birth)

You will get cramps after delivery that feel similar to menstrual cramps. The afterpains are caused by uterine contractions as are menstrual cramps. These cramps tend to be more common in second pregnancies or in women over 35. The cramps may increase during nursing because the hormone oxytocin will stimulate the uterus to contract even more. These cramps are nothing to worry about and are a sign that all is "shrinking" well.

Black and blue all over

Occasionally, broken blood vessels in your face, caused by straining and pushing, will make you look like you're auditioning for the next *Rocky* flick. This is a normal postpartum symptom that will heal. Your eyes may look bloodshot, and you may have black and blue marks under your eyes (caused by healing and drainage). You may also have bruises or tiny red dots on your face and upper chest area. Cold compresses—and time—will heal all wounds.

Bladder problems

You may have difficulty emptying your bladder and may also feel as though it is burning when you urinate. The burning sensation is caused by urine hitting sensitive vaginal tears or incisions. Some women also have difficulty sensing that their bladders are full, which is caused by a numb bladder from bruising or trauma during delivery, or even by anesthetic medications that interfere with urinary "signals." Normal bladder sensation usually returns very quickly. Some women may need a catheter. If, however, urinary problems persist, you may have developed a urinary tract infection, discussed in detail in chapter 3. It's also important to make an effort to empty your bladder as soon as you can after delivery and about every six hours thereafter. This keeps the bladder in shape and helps prevent UTIs. After about 24 hours, you'll be urinating frequently again as your body begins to empty out all the excess fluid of pregnancy.

If you're breastfeeding, these bladder problems may persist as a result of a lower estrogen level but will be greatly helped by something known as the Kegel exercise. This is a very convenient exercise that you can do in any position, anywhere, anytime: in an elevator, on the subway in a movie theater, or while you're cooking, eating, or lying down. All you do is isolate the muscle that stops and starts your urinary stream. You can also insert your finger into your vagina and try to squeeze your vaginal opening around your finger. Once you've isolated the muscle, just squeeze five times, then release and count to five; and squeeze again. Or, squeeze 10 and count 10. You can also do the exercise by stopping and starting your stream every time you urinate. Either Kegel method is fine, so long as you keep doing it. The key is to keep the muscles in shape. Its that simple, and it really helps. You can also do general exercises to firm up your abdomen and pelvis in conjunction with your Kegel exercises.

Bleeding

As the uterus shrinks back to normal, the lining will expel itself. You'll be bleeding anywhere from two to six weeks after delivery. This bleeding is known as lochia and is your uterus's way of emptying out all its "gunk"—for lack of a better word. A major part of the bleeding is also due to the healing of the former site of your placenta.

The bleeding will start out as bright red and then will change to a menstrual flow consistency. It later changes into a pink, watery flow, ending in a yellowish discharge. If you're breastfeeding, the hormone oxytocin may cause your uterus to contract more intensely, which in turn may cause the flow to become brighter and bloodier each time you nurse. Sometimes the contractions help to reduce the flow, which will mean that some women will notice that the flow subsides when they breastfeed. Either case is normal. The uterine contractions are your body's way of pinching off blood vessels and preventing hemorrhaging.

If your bleeding is heavy, meaning that you need to change a full-size maxi-pad every hour, you should contact your doctor immediately. This may be a sign that you're experiencing a postpartum hemorrhage, where a piece of the placenta is left behind in your uterus. If this is the case, you may need a D & C. Postpartum hemorrhaging is discussed in detail towards the end of this chapter.

Bowels

You'll probably be constipated for a few days after delivery. What you need is a salad, lots of bran, and *People* magazine. While some women liken pushing during labor to having a bowel movement, others liken the first postpartum bowel movement to pushing out a baby! It's painful, and it hurts!

As for the physical reasons that interfere with bowel function, the abdominal muscles that bring down your stools may have been stretched out during childbirth, causing them to be a bit out of shape. They will repair themselves eventually, though. Sometimes the bowel itself has been traumatized by childbirth and may not be up to snuff. Finally, you may have already emptied it during childbirth and simply not have eaten enough for it to have "refilled."

The remedies are repetitive and boring but include roughage and fiber, plenty of fluids, and a little exercise (a stroll down the hall is fine for starters). Kegel exercises will be helpful in getting your muscles back in shape. You should also avoid straining, not because your stitches will tear, but because it will aggravate your hemorrhoids. Review chapters 3 and 4 for more information on constipation.

Breasts

Your breasts will undergo the most radical changes at this stage, particularly as they become engorged with milk and you begin breast-feeding. See chapter 9 for everything you want to know about breasts, nipples, and breastfeeding.

Edema (fluid retention)

During delivery, you lose a great deal of fluid. Ironically, this can cause *more* fluid retention. The reason has to do with the shifting of your fluid levels. General puffiness is common, but your legs and ankles in particular might become swollen for a few days after delivery. Watching your salt intake and elevating your feet may be helpful. If your legs and ankles remain swollen for more than a week after delivery, your doctor may prescribe a diuretic; this will greatly depend on whether you're breastfeeding, however.

Hair loss

Some women become alarmed about an apparent hair loss after delivery, characterized by huge clumps of hair falling out when they brush it. This is absolutely normal and is caused by hormonal shifts in your body. Some women do not experience what should be a normal hair loss during pregnancy. When they don't, the body "comes to collect," balancing out the hair loss "requirements." To do this, it takes out the hair you should have lost throughout the last nine months all in one clump, making the hair loss more obvious. You're not going bald, you don't need a wig, and your hair production will resume shortly.

Hemorrhoids

This should really be called "The Things That Wouldn't Leave." If you managed to escape hemorrhoids so far, they may plague you after delivery. All that pushing puts tremendous pressure on the rectal area, causing hemorrhoids. If you already had hemorrhoids at the time of delivery, they'll get worse. Just grin and bear it. These are very common after delivery, but they will get better. Review chapters 3 and 4 for more information about hemorrhoidal treatment.

Menstrual cycles

If you're breastfeeding, you most likely won't get your period anywhere from 4 to 6 months after delivery regardless of whether the child is weaned. Some women don't get their periods until after they've weaned. However, many women will continue to ovulate while they breastfeed, which is why pregnancy is a risk. About 50% of all women who breastfeed ovulate by the 12th postpartum week, while roughly 50% of all women who bottlefeed will ovulate in the 6th postpartum week. So beware and make sure you use contraception, discussed further below.

Pains in the butt

Pain, numbness, and general soreness around your entire vaginal/ perineal area is a consequence of childbirth. Whether you've had an episiotomy or a perfectly natural vaginal delivery, soreness will persist for a few days, making walking and sitting comfortably seem difficult. An ice pack for a few days after delivery can help swelling and discomfort. (Besides, you'll be so busy, you may not even notice!)

Perspiring in buckets

First, make sure you're not running a fever, which can be a sign of infection. When that's ruled out, relax! You are literally sweating out the eau de pregnancy fluids that you've been retaining for the last three fiscal quarters. This may go on for several weeks. Just wear loose clothing and deodorant. You may also want to keep a towel over your pillow to absorb the sweat at night. If heart palpitations, extreme irritability, an intolerance to heat, or a buggy/stary look in your eyes accompanies the sweating, request a thyroid function test. Your excessive perspiration may be caused by hyperthyroidism (overactive thyroid gland), discussed more in chapter 2. Generally, this is a concern only if thyroid disorders run in your family.

Skin changes

You'll start to get your own skin colors back! Your darkened nipples, darkened vulva, and linea negra (that dark line running from abdomen to the pubic line) will fade. And remember those spidery lines on your chest, neck, and shoulders? They'll disappear too.

Stretch marks

Yes, it's true, you will get these. The stretching and tearing of your skin's elastic fibers will leave stretch marks over the most "stretched out" areas: your abdomen, breasts, thighs, and buttocks. While the stretch marks may have been red and rather unsightly during pregnancy, after delivery they will begin to fade, changing to a silvery color but never completely disappearing.

Warning Signs

It's difficult to distinguish normal discomforts from unusual symptoms that warrant immediate medical attention, so here's a warning list. If you develop *any* of the following symptoms, call your doctor immediately. In severe cases follow the emergency procedures outlined at the end of chapter 3.

- Heavy bleeding (indicates a possible hemorrhage).
- Blood clots that are the size of lemons or larger (indicates the placenta hasn't completely expelled).
- Sharp pains in your chest (indicates a possible blood clot in your lungs).
- Persistent fever either by itself or in conjunction with abdominal or breast pain (breast pain + fever = bacterial breast infection; fever + abdominal pain = pelvic infection).
- Foul smelling discharge (spells I-N-F-E-C-T-I-O-N).
- Difficulty urinating or painful urination (indicates possible UTI, discussed in chapter 3).
- Extremely tender breasts or an isolated red area or tender area on the breast (spells I-N-F-E-C-T-I-O-N).
- Swollen red area on your leg (may indicate a blood clot).
- Extreme depression (see chapter 10 on postpartum depression).

Weight loss

You'll begin losing your "baby fat" at this stage, particularly if you breastfeed. According to a study published in the Journal of the American Dietetic Association, breastfeeding "officially" causes a more rapid weight loss, seen particularly in the lower body area. This weight loss does not happen overnight, however. It takes several weeks for your uterus to shrink back to its normal size. If you had a normal vaginal delivery, Kegel exercises will help to tighten your muscles as well. If you're breastfeeding, it's imperative that you do not diet until baby is weaned! You'll need to keep up your caloric intake in order to produce high-quality milk. (See chapter 9 for more details.)

If You've Had an Episiotomy

Whether you've had an all-out episiotomy or have been stitched up because you've torn your perineum (the area between your anus and vagina), you'll feel swollen and sore. Sneezing and coughing may also aggravate the pain. Intercourse is out of the question until your stitches have been removed (or have dissolved), and your doctor gives the final okay. Once your episiotomy has healed, sexual intercourse shouldn't hurt, but the area around the healed episiotomy may feel tight, tender, or prickly. The vagina may also feel dry because your low estrogen levels will decrease the amount of the vaginal lubrication usually felt during intercourse (discussed below). If painful intercourse persists, you should definitely see your doctor and try to pin down why you're still in pain.

Sitz baths (very shallow baths that just barely cover your rear end) are recommended if you've had an episiotomy. The warmth will increase blood flow to the area, help clean the area, and speed up healing. Since sitting comfortably may be difficult, you can use an inflatable doughnut to sit on for the first few days. If you like, you can also apply cold packs to the scar, which will help keep it from swelling.

If pain around your scar persists after your stitches have been removed, let your doctor know. Your scar may have become infected. Keeping the incision very clean is the best way to help the incision heal. If the scar has become infected for some reason, you'll be prescribed an antibiotic.

Some practitioners may recommend Kegel exercises at this point, most of you will not be able to do Kegels until your episiotomy stitches have healed. Don't feel guilty about avoiding Kegels for a while.

If You've Had a Cesarean Section

The good news is that you will not be suffering any perineal/vaginal discomfort like your vaginal delivery friends, so you'll be able to sit comfortably and walk around with a little more ease. Your bowel movements may also be less painful, but you'll still suffer from the fear of tearing stitches as well as from constipation. You'll also experience bleeding, afterpains, and the rest of the symptoms listed above.

On top of this, you'll be recovering from major abdominal surgery, which means that the entire area from your waist down may feel numb. This numbness may interfere with urinating and defecating, but will wear off in a few hours. Depending on how severe your urinary or bowel problems are, catheters, stool softeners, and even enemas may be recommended.

If you've had a spinal anesthetic, you'll need to lie flat on your back for about 8–12 hours, but you'll still be able to breastfeed and bond with your baby. If you've had a general anesthetic, you may have a reaction to the drugs and may be vomiting or just feel nauseous. This is normal and is nothing to worry about.

Once the anesthetic wears off, you'll begin to feel some pain around the incision just above your pubic line. Again, what one woman finds extremely painful, another finds mildly uncomfortable. Pain relief medication will be prescribed as needed. Digestive problems may persist for a couple of days after the anesthetic wears off because surgery has interfered with your digestive tract. This causes gas, which can feel very uncomfortable, particularly if pressure is put on your scar line. Speak to your doctor if the gas pains are intolerable. Getting up and going for a walk is the best remedy.

You can expect to be home in less than a week, and your stitches will be removed within that time frame. Some stitches just absorb into the skin, which means that you may be sent home even earlier. Review the warning list above, and watch for signs of fever, particularly accompanied by abdominal discomfort. This is a sign that you may have a pelvic infection caused by bacteria entering your pelvic tract during surgery.

If You've Had a High-Risk Pregnancy

Whether you've had twins, developed gestational diabetes or gestational hypertension, or have a chronic health condition, your postpartum state will not differ from that of any other woman. However, you may have more severe symptoms, and may require extra care and treatment after the birth. For example, after a multiple birth, afterpains and bleeding may be more severe or persist for longer periods of time, while bowel and bladder disruption may be more severe.

If you have another illness, gestational or chronic, you'll need to be seen by both your obstetrician and the specialist who manages your condition. You may require certain foods, vitamin supplements, or medications after delivery. All these will vary depending on your condition.

Postpartum Sex

Childbirth practitioners advise that even with a normal vaginal delivery, intercourse should be avoided for about 4–6 weeks after delivery, for the reasons discussed at the beginning of this chapter. Again, if you had a cesarean section or episiotomy, you must heal properly to avoid feeling extreme pain or ripping your stitches. Until intercourse resumes, you can manually or orally stimulate your partner. (You're probably not going to be interested yourself, however.)

Almost all surveys done on postpartum sexuality report that fatigue is the most common barrier to lovemaking. A little honesty, sensitivity, and communication between yourself and your partner goes a long way. When intercourse resumes, it will not be the same as it was prior to the pregnancy. First, if you're breastfeeding, your adjusting hormone levels will interfere with your libido even further, and you may not have the same level of desire. Second, your lower estrogen levels interfere with vaginal lubrication, which means that you'll need to use a synthetic lubricant. You may also need to adjust your positions to accommodate a sore perineal area. A "woman on top" or side-entry position may be a good idea, which can allow you to guide the penis and insert it at your own speed.

The most drastic change in your sex life will be caused by your vagina. Unfortunately, childbirth does stretch the vagina, and it never goes back to its nice, taut, prepregnant tension. This may dramatically change the sensation for you and your partner, as the grip will not be as tight as it once was.

Don't despair, however. Kegel exercises will help (again, these may be difficult if you've had an episiotomy). Abdominal exercises will also help tighten your muscles as well as improve your own body image. The best trick is to use your fingers during intercourse to simulate that prepregnancy grip. Here's how to do it: Get into a hands-free intercourse position and manually close your vaginal lips around the base of the penis during thrusting. This will improve matters tremendously. As frustrating as your new vagina may feel to you, please don't consider surgery to tighten it up unless there is a good medical reason that warrants it.

A Word About Breastfeeding "Arousal"

As you may know or may have heard, you can get sexually aroused when you breastfeed. The uterus literally contracts each time the baby nurses, which tends to stimulate your vagina and clitoris. Don't be embarrassed by this or feel as though you're a sexual deviant. Many women feel the need to masturbate (or have sex with their partner) after feeding. Many women also find that the nipple stimulation is arousing because, after all, the nipple is a sexual organ in and of itself. Finally, breastfeeding may make you feel fabulously feminine and maternal, which many women find a turn-on. The worst thing you can do is deny yourself these feelings. Pregnancy, childbearing and feeding are all sexual processes that stimulate every sexual impulse within you. In fact, the arousal women feel from breastfeeding may be why breastfeeding was unpopular in the conservative years of the 1950s and 1960s.

Contraception

No, breastfeeding does *not* offer 100% contraceptive protection. And the rhythm method is totally out of the question since you haven't a clue when your next menstrual cycle will come. If you're having sex, you must have protected sex unless you don't mind doing the whole thing all over again. Childbirth practitioners recommend that you wait a couple of years between pregnancies to give your body a chance to recuperate. Your calcium levels will need to rebalance as well as your hemoglobin levels. Your energy levels have been enormously depleted as well, and should be given a rest.

If you're breastfeeding, the best method of contraception is a condom with spermicide. Then you can graduate to a barrier method such as a diaphragm, cervical cap, or vaginal sponge. Oral contraceptives that contain estrogen may alter the composition of breast milk, but hormonal contraceptives that are progesterone-only, such as Norplant or Depo-Provera, are fine if you're breastfeeding and don't alter the milk in any way. Barrier methods are very safe and pose fewer risks to you. However, unless barrier methods are combined with spermicide and a condom, they offer no protection against STDs.

If you're not breastfeeding, you can go on hormonal contraceptives shortly after delivery or use a barrier method. IUDs cannot be inserted immediately after childbirth because the risk of infection is too high. If you really want to use an IUD at this stage, discuss the risks with your doctor and make sure you're making an informed decision. Otherwise, waiting until the uterus shrinks back to its normal size (anywhere from 6-8 weeks or longer) is necessary before you're refitted for an IUD.

Finally, if you don't want any more children, you may be an excellent candidate for *tubal ligation,* also known as permanent contraception. Discuss this option with your doctor.

Diaphragms

If you already have a diaphragm, throw it away now! You need to be refitted for a new diaphragm following childbirth. You'll also need to wait a few weeks before you vagina shrinks to its new size. For those of you who have never used a diaphragm it's a dome-shaped cup with a flexible rim that fits over your cervix and rests behind your pubic bone. It looks like a tiny rubber flying saucer. It's inserted before intercourse, and blocks the sperm from entering the uterus through the cervix. The failure rate ranges from 10% to 20%. This is considerably higher than hormonal methods, but much of the failure has to do with improper use and insertion. Diaphragms come in different sizes and styles. You'll need to be fitted for one by either your family doctor or gynecologist. Once you're fitted, you'll be given a prescription, and you can purchase the diaphragm at any drugstore, or your own doctor may dispense it as his or her office. Then, you'll need to go back to your doctor and be shown how to use it yourself. Sometimes you'll need a plastic inserter. Go home and practice and see your doctor one more time before you use it, so he or she can make sure you're putting it in correctly. Before your doctor recommends a diaphragm, he or she should perform a pelvic exam to make sure that you don't have any physical abnormalities that would prevent you from using one in the first place. It's important to get a diaphragm that fits well; if it's too small, it will expose the cervix; if it's too big, it will buckle. You must be refitted if you've gained or lost more than 15 pounds, had pelvic surgery, had another child, or had an abortion or miscarriage.

Your diaphragm shouldn't interfere with normal activities. Urination or bowel movements shouldn't be affected, and you should be able to bathe and shower normally. If it is interfering with these activities, it may not be in properly or might be the wrong size.

Cervical caps

Cervical caps must also be refitted after childbirth. The cervical cap is a small, thimble-shaped cap that blocks only the cervix and not the entire upper part of the vaginal canal the way a diaphragm does. In essence, the cervical cap is a mini-diaphragm with a tall dome. You simply insert the cap with your forefinger and place it over the cervix yourself. About 6% of cervical cap candidates will not be able to find one that fits (shorter or longer cervices are a problem, apparently).

Vaginal contraceptive sponges

Also known as the sponge, the vaginal sponge, and the contraceptive sponge, this is such a simple, easy-to-use, and effective product, it's shocking that it has only been available since 1983. It looks like a cap made out of thick sponge material, and it's designed to fit inside the upper vagina with its concave side covering the cervix. If you imagine a catchers mitt, the open glove side faces the cervix; the back of the glove faces the vaginal opening. It even has a little loop attached to it that you just pull on to remove it. Although failure rates run slightly higher (17%–24%), the sponge can be purchased over-the-counter. You don't need to be fitted! The sponge is individually wrapped for onetime use only, like a condom. It also comes with built-in spermicide. The only sponge on the market right now is called the Today Sponge. It's slightly pillow-shaped, made out of polyurethane, and contains nonoxynol-9 spermicide. You can use this once your cervix has closed up again.

When Something Goes Wrong

Although something can go wrong with your newborn following childbirth, this book does not attempt to cover any of these issues. This section deals with problems that can occur in your body following childbirth. For books on neonatal care, review Appendix B at the back of this book.

Postpartum Hemorrhage

This means that the normal bleeding that follows childbirth is heavier than normal, may contain clots, and is uncontrolled. A foul smell may also accompany the bleeding, which indicates that an infection is the culprit. When bright red discharge persists after about the fourth day following delivery, this may also indicate a hemorrhage. In the past, this was a common cause of maternal death following childbirth. Today, very few women die from a postpartum hemorrhage in North America.

There are two kinds of postpartum hemorrhage. Immediate and late. Immediate postpartum hemorrhage is commonly caused by *uterine atony*, where the uterus fails to contract normally after delivery. The uterus must contract in order to control the bleeding and pinch off blood vessels. Women who are most prone to uterine atony after childbirth are those who:

- had a long, exhausting labor and/or delivery;
- had a traumatic delivery;
- had an abnormally distended uterus because of a multiple birth, excess amniotic fluid, or a large baby (in this case, the uterus isn't able to contract enough to accommodate the distention);
- had a placenta that separated prematurely (see chapter 6);
- had an odd-shaped placenta;
- have fibroids that are interfering with normal uterine contractions;
- have a condition such as anemia or toxemia that is interfering with healing; or
- have blood clotting abnormalities.

Other causes of immediate postpartum hemorrhage can be lacerations that don't heal, which occur during childbirth. These lacerations can be anywhere—in the uterus, cervix, vagina, and so on—and can cause hemorrhaging immediately following delivery as well.

Retained placental tissue within the uterus is a third cause, while a pelvic infection (discussed next) is a fourth.

When the placenta expels, sometimes the uterus is turned inside out, like a sleeve. This is called a *uterine rupture,* and is a common cause of hemorrhaging immediately following delivery.

Late postpartum hemorrhage (as late as two weeks after delivery) is caused most often by retained placental tissue. Late hemorrhaging could also result if the placental site doesn't heal after delivery, called a *subinvolution.* And finally, a pelvic infection (discussed next) can cause late postpartum hemorrhaging.

How is it treated?

The first thing most practitioners will do is massage your uterus to encourage contractions. If that doesn't work, you may be given drugs that will trigger uterine contractions, such as oxytocin or synthetic prostaglandin. If that fails, your doctor will then try to find the cause—retained placental tissue or a laceration—and either manually repair the laceration or remove the placental tissue via D & C.

If bleeding remains uncontrolled, you will be given fluids intravenously and perhaps a blood-clotting medication. If absolutely every attempt was made to control the bleeding and it's still out of control, the very last resort may be a hysterectomy. If this is the case, make sure every effort was made to control the bleeding, discuss all other options and the consequences and risks of each option, and don't consent to a hysterectomy unless you feel comfortable with the decision.

Bacterial Infections

Normally, the cervix acts as a barrier to bacteria and prevents them from getting inside the upper pelvic region. But when the cervix dilates as much as it does during childbirth, bacteria can enter the uterus and do a lot of damage. A bacterial infection can spread higher inside your uterus and cause infection of the uterine lining or uterine muscle. This can result in an inflammation of the uterine lining (known as *endometritis*—not to be confused with endometriosis!) or inflammation of the uterine muscle (known as *myometritis*). You're also vulnerable to infection after a miscarriage, therapeutic abortion, D & C, and even amniocentesis.

These infections are different from PID (Pelvic Inflammatory Disease), which is mainly caused by chlamydia, gonorrhea, and IUD usage. The bacteria that cause endometritis or myometritis in this case is usually a streptococcus, bacteria that normally inhabit the vagina. If you've recently been infected with an STD after childbirth, however, you are at a higher risk for developing PID.

The symptoms can really vary depending on what is infected. The most common symptom is lower abdominal pain due to uterine tenderness. This may be accompanied by a high fever and foul-smelling vaginal discharge, which may contain pus. Sometimes the pain is present when you urinate or move your bowels.

Other symptoms include lower back pain, nausea and dizziness, low fever, chills, abnormal bleeding, frequent urination, a burning sensation during urination or an inability to empty the bladder, feeling like you have to constantly move your bowels, a general feeling of ill health, and abdominal bloating.

Diagnosing infections

Pain and fever are the most common symptoms, which should make your doctor suspect infection. First, a general physical exam will be done to check for other problems (respiratory, for example). Then, an abdominal and pelvic exam will be done. If you had either an episiotomy or cesarean section, your incision scars will be examined and appropriate cultures will be obtained.

Sometimes an ultrasound test is helpful. It can show whether your pelvic organs are inflamed or whether an abscess has developed on any of the organs. A blood sample can show whether you have an elevated white blood cell count, a sign of infection.

Treating a bacterial infection

Once your infection is diagnosed, successful treatment is based on identifying the right bacteria responsible for the infection in the first place. You may need further blood tests for this. Once the right bacteria are identified, an appropriate antibiotic will be prescribed. Depending on the severity of your infection, you may need to receive antibiotic therapy intravenously. You may need to stop breastfeeding during treatment, because some antibiotics cannot be taken if you're breastfeeding.

The general medication regimen involves intravenous antibiotics for two days, or until the pain and fever are gone. Then, you may be given antibiotics to take orally for a week or so, after you're home. Depending on the cause of infection, a follow-up culture may be necessary. Surgery is seldom necessary to treat a postpartum bacterial infection, but occasionally, abscesses may form, and will therefore need to be drained. It's also possible for these infections to involve the fallopian tubes, which could result in a future fertility problem. Make sure to ask your doctor whether you are at risk for this.

Taking care of yourself after childbirth is essential for your health as well as your newborn's health and well-being. The healthier you are, the healthier your breast milk will be, and the more energy you'll have for feeding and nurturing. If you're not breastfeeding, you'll still need lots of energy to care for your newborn, which can happen only if you've taken care of yourself. In fact, whether you're breastfeeding or bottle-feeding, the next chapter will help you make the breastfeeding decision, while discussing all of the changes your breasts will undergo, breastfeeding or not.

9

Breasts, Feeding, and Other Milk "Beefs"

*"Oh God—my body's making milk! It's like waking up one day
to discover you can get bacon out of your elbow!"*
—courtesy MURPHY BROWN

I like the above quote because it essentially describes how breast milk, whether you choose to breastfeed or not, changes your perception of yourself. You're now a nurturer, someone capable of giving food and sustenance to another human being. When you stop and think about it, this is a rather fantastic accomplishment.

Breastfeeding, of course, also changes your *body!* That's why I've not only devoted an entire chapter to this subject, but have written *The Breastfeeding Sourcebook,* which was inspired by this chapter. The purpose here is not only to give you all the information you need about engorgement, getting started, feeding techniques, and diet, but also to discuss the more common problems that revolve around breastfeeding. These problems include breast infections, nipple infections, and an inadequate milk supply (often due to inadequate information). And because as a result of pregnancy your breasts will have changed in appearance and will change again after you wean your baby, this chapter discusses BSE—Breast Self Examination—something *all* women 35 and over must be vigilant about as their bodies age. Unfortunately, as wondrous as the breast is, it is also vulnerable to cancer. Ninety percent of all breast cancers are found through BSE, discussed at the end of this chapter.

This chapter also discusses the health implications, practical considerations, and "political" issues surrounding the breastfeeding versus bottle-feeding debate. My intent is to provide you with a balanced approach so you can make an informed decision. Finally, I've included an overall breast refresher course, discussing how breasts work, something you should know if you're going to use them. However, for an expansive look at breastfeeding, please consult my book *The Breastfeeding Sourcebook*.

Breasts 101

Normally, when we think of our reproductive organs, we think only of our pelvic contents, which consist of the uterus, fallopian tubes, and ovaries. But the breasts are an integral part of our reproductive system. The sole, technical purpose of breasts is to produce milk to feed a baby. In fact, it is the breasts that define our biological class: the word mammal comes from the term mammary glands. Although mammal breasts vary in size and number, we are the only biological group that breastfeeds. However, the difference between human females and other animals is that we are the only ones who develop full breasts long before they're needed for breastfeeding. This has to do with our sexual behavior. Since primates are also the only kind of animals that engage in sex when they are not necessarily fertile, the breasts serve a very important sexual purpose as well. As discussed in chapters 4, 6, and 8, nipple stimulation releases oxytocin, the hormone that not only triggers milk let down (see below), but uterine contractions, which researchers say enhances sexual sensation.

Human breast tissue begins to develop in the sixth week of fetal life. The milk ridge, a line from the armpit all the way down to the groin, develops at this point. By the ninth week in most cases, the milk ridge has reached the chest area, but both women and men can develop accessory nipples and even breast tissue all the way down to the groin. These will look like moles to the untrained eye. But other mammals retain the milk ridge, which is the reason why they have multiple nipples. When you're born, then, you already have breast tissue, as does your own newborn. And since the mother's sex hormones have been circulating throughout the placenta, both boys and girls are born with little breasts. Your newborn may even have nipple discharge. This is known as "witch's milk" and goes away in a couple of weeks as the baby is weaned from your hormones. Between 80 and 90% of newborns have this discharge the second or third day after birth.

For women, nothing much happens to the breast until puberty, when the pituitary gland starts the entire reproductive and development cycle. Puberty is triggered by follicle-stimulating hormone (FSH), estrogen, and progesterone and includes the development of pubic hair and so forth. Young girls will usually sprout breast buds prior to pubic hair, but it could happen the other way around.

Breasts begin to develop at this point, and their development consists of five stages. The prepubertal stage is when the nipple becomes slightly more prominent; the breast bud stage is the beginning of breast development. The third stage, breast elevation, is when the breast is formed and more erect; the fourth stage, the areolar mound, is when the areola enlarges in circumference. At the final stage, the adult contour, the breast is mature enough to produce milk. Breasts are considered mature when they are capable of breastfeeding. The menstrual period is usually the "finale" to the breast's development.

The Pregnant and Postpartum Breast

The breasts are prepared for pregnancy each month. Estrogen causes the increase of ductal tissue in the breast, while progesterone causes the increase in lobular tissue. The result is swollen, sometimes painful breasts, which subside as the menstrual cycle comes to an end.

During pregnancy, the breasts enlarge rapidly and become firm. The little glands around the areola (the dark skin surrounding the nipple) known as Montgomery's glands become darker and more prominent. The areola itself gets even darker, and the nipples become larger and more erect, preparing themselves for future milk production. There are two main hormones responsible for milk production: prolactin and oxytocin, which are also responsible for triggering postpartum uterine contractions. Both are released by the pituitary gland, which is stimulated by an area of the brain known as the hypothalamus. Prolactin is sometimes called the mothering hormone and is crucial for breastfeeding; without it, you can't make milk. Prolactin goes to work around the eighth week of pregnancy, and its levels rise for the next seven months, peaking at your baby's birth. At this point, your body is also producing high levels of estrogen and progesterone, which block some of the prolactin receptors and inhibit milk production. Once the baby is born, your levels of estrogen and progesterone drop very quickly, while the prolactin levels drop at a far slower and almost unnoticeable rate. You now begin to produce milk, and breastfeeding can begin. At first, a premilk substance known as *colostrum* comes out, which nourishes the baby until the actual breast milk comes. Colostrum is now being looked upon in a new light by researchers as we discover some truly amazing ingredients. These include factors that activate bowel function, complex immunological proteins, and living white blood cells. Many women will leak colostrum during pregnancy (discussed in chapter 4).

Your Milk Delivery System

Your baby would not get enough milk if weren't for oxytocin. Oxytocin is responsible for milk delivery or "let down." The baby's sucking not only brings out the milk but sends a message to the pituitary gland via the nipples' nerve endings (the thoracic nerves) and the hypothalamus, to send down the milk. The pituitary gland responds by manufacturing oxytocin, which makes the tiny muscles lining your breasts contract and spray milk out from the nipple. So while some of the milk is actually sucked out by the baby, a lot of the milk just squirts down the baby's throat. The breast is just about the only organ in the reproductive system that works on *supply and demand*. The suckling triggers more milk; the lack of regular suckling inhibits milk production. An inadequate milk supply often has more to do with not learning how to properly suckle your newborn than with a failing to produce enough milk.

In the days of wet nurses, aristocratic mothers would not breast-feed because they were considered too frail to produce good milk. Instead, a wet nurse would breastfeed the baby. Wet nurses stayed "wet" by continually breastfeeding after they themselves had children. In effect, one could conceivably breastfeed for years; as long as the suckling is there, the breast milk will continue.

The Breast Rehearsal

The problem is, not all newborns know instinctively how to suckle. This is the case after a hard birth, with a newborn who is ill, tongue-tied, has a small chin or cleft lip/palate, or who has perhaps been thumb-sucking in utero. External factors can also create nipple confusion, such as mothers with inverted nipples, nipple scarring from previous breast surgery, or ignorant healthcare providers who introduce artificial nipples to the newborn. You have to show your baby how to suckle, by essentially having a breastfeeding rehearsal. Unfortunately, many new mothers aren't aware of this fact. When their initial breastfeeding attempts end in dismal failure, they feel as though their breasts just "weren't made for suckling." As a result, many of these women give up and decide that bottlefeeding is the only route. This is a most unfortunate choice that has more to do with poor lactation counseling than poor lactation!

Several days of bumbling breastfeeding attempts is the rule, not the exception. Every woman can breastfeed, but some women will have more obstacles than others. With the appropriate instruction, most moth-

ers who want to breastfeed will be able to. What you may need is a referral to a board-certified lactation consultant (LC), usually a public health
nurse or midwife who specializes in assisting mothers and newborns
with lactation. (Many obstetricians and family practitioners will also do
this.) While all hospitals in North America today should have these consultants on staff, many don't. If they don't, your doctor or midwife can
give you the name of one. Or, you can contact your local chapter of the
La Leche League, an association made up of breastfeeding advocates,
listed in the White Pages. You can also refer to appendix A in this book.

It's crucial to note that only about 1% of all mothers are biologi-
cally incapable of producing enough breast milk for their newborns. Yet
as any lactation consultant will testify, even these women can maintain a
partial breast milk supply, which can be supplemented by formula or donated breast milk. There are also medications, known as *lactogogues,*
which can increase milk production if you have a lagging milk supply. If
you need to supplement your milk because of the baby's health, this can
be done by slipping a small feeding tube along side the nipple when the
baby is finished feeding. This will keep up breast stimulation and milk
production, while supplementing by bottle will reduce breastmilk production. If you must miss a nursing for any reason, you can express milk
via pump to keep up production. Here are some important "getting
started" tips:

- Do not allow anyone to supplement your feedings with sugar
  water or formula unless there is a good medical reason! Make
  your objections to this practice very clear on your birth plan.
  (Few hospitals have abandoned this practice, however, so you
  may need to be aggressive about this objection.)
- Don't introduce your newborn to any false nipples, such as
  pacifiers (soothers) or bottles. Lactation consultants recommend allowing at least 6 weeks of good breastfeeding to pass
  before introducing a pacifier. Artificial nipples require your
  baby to learn a tongue-thrust habit referred to as 'nipple confusion.' This will not only prevent effective nursing but will
  make hamburger out of your nipple.

- If your baby is "tongue tied," when he or she cries, the tongue rises up in a heart shape instead of a smooth curve. The fold of tissue under the tongue will need to be clipped. (Ask your lactation consultant or pediatrician about where to get this done.)
- Never wear nipple shields while breastfeeding. These not only cause nipple confusion, but also block nipple stimulation, which is necessary for adequate milk production.
- Educate yourself about breastfeeding before the birth. Attend a La Leche meeting, consult with an LC, read, and so on!
- Plan to nurse at least ten times a day (about every two hours during daylight) and about every 3 hours during the night. This will prevent engorgement, bring the milk in sooner, and prevent jaundice in the baby.

Feeding instructions

The first rule about breastfeeding is: ASAP. Babies tend to be more alert and interested in feeding in the first hour following birth. You should begin to feed in the delivery room as soon as your baby's health signs are pronounced "strong" (see chapter 7 for details) unless there is a good reason not to. If you intend to breastfeed from the outset, you might want to list your desire to *immediately* breastfeed on your birth plan (also discussed in chapter 7). Here are the step-by-step instructions:

STEP 1: Tummy-to-tummy. Once you're in a comfortable sitting position, position your baby with its tummy to yours. Your body should be level. Manually pull out your nipple (with your thumb and index finger) so that it is erect. Bring your baby to your breast rather than the breast to the baby.

STEP 2: Nose-to-nipple. The baby's nose should be level with your nipple. Don't block the baby's nose with your own breast! Support your breast by placing four fingers underneath it, away from the areola, with your thumb on the nipple (the "c-hold").

STEP 3: Tickle 'til wide-open mouth. Now take the nipple and lightly brush the baby's lips with it. This will get the baby interested, and may trigger its instinct to suckle. It will also make the nipple erect. Do this until the baby opens his or her mouth wide. Aim the nipple into the center of the baby's mouth. You can even arouse your baby's sense of taste and smell by expressing a few drops of milk. You'll need to repeat this step *several times* before you can move on to step 4. You can move on to step 4, once the baby takes the nipple into its mouth. Do NOT force the nipple in; this will "turn off" the baby.

STEP 4: Pop baby on! Make sure the baby takes the areola into its mouth along with the nipple. This is very crucial. Sucking on a nipple alone will cause soreness and cracking. It is the areola that contains the milk glands. Unless this is being suckled, your milk delivery system will break down. When you see the baby taking the nipple, pull him or her toward you quickly, which will encourage a better grip and help the baby's tongue and lips close over the area.

STEP 5: Check the latch. Your baby is latched on properly if the mouth is widely open around the breast; the tip of the tongue is above the lower lip and is cradled around your nipple; the nose is just touching the breast. In addition, the jaw should be moving up and down, the ears wiggle, and the nipple feels COMFORTABLE. Cheeks should NOT be sucking in and out as they do with bottlefeeding.

STEP 6: When your baby is "full" and has clearly stopped feeding, *don't* pull out the nipple yet. Make sure your baby isn't still latched on by putting your finger into the baby's mouth to let in some air, which helps the baby let go. You can also just press down on your breast and help to pull back the nipple.

The Milkman Cometh: Engorgement

You should begin to breastfeed before your milk "comes in" to help prevent engorgement, which means to be "overfilled" with milk. Although most doctors will tell you that engorgement is normal, lactation consultants maintain that it's caused by poor breastfeeding management, poor latch, and/or not feeding often or long enough. In other words, with proper instruction after birth, engorgement is preventable. In fact, it's better to start before you become engorged because the engorgement can be painful and may cause the nipple to be swollen and hence "flat." The pain of engorgement is caused by an increased blood supply to the breast combined with an accumulation of milk. This spells trouble for the breastfeeding novice and can frustrate the baby, who may have an incredible instinct to suckle. When the initial feeding is delayed anywhere from 24 to 36 hours after birth, you may be forced to feed after you're engorged, which is why ASAP is the rule!

Why feed the baby when the milk isn't there yet? Well, the best answer has to with establishing a "just in time" delivery system. You're not just a mother and nurturer, you're also a manufacturer. But since you manufacture milk for only one customer, you can't afford to lose any product. So you'll need to make sure that the product is ready to be delivered just in time.

To develop a "just in time" strategy, you need to beat the milk by a few days by feeding your baby "premilk," or colostrum, until about the third or fourth postpartum day. The colostrum is like a product "sample" that will keep the customer satisfied until the stock comes in. Then, by the time your milk comes in, the baby's mouth will be there to accept the milk, which will help to alleviate the feeling of fullness and extreme discomfort that engorgement can cause. As your colostrum decreases, your milk may look thin and watery. You may also feel a tingling sensation in your breasts as your milk begins "letting down."

Essentially, engorgement feels exactly like it sounds: engorged, meaning congested and overfilled. Milk may leak out of your breasts and spill down your shirt, and if you're not wearing a proper nursing bra, your shirts may become soaked with breast milk. Breast pads are available to wear inside your bra. Your breasts and armpit area will feel swollen, hard, and sore, and you may wish to use ice packs for the first few days of engorgement. Happily, engorgement is only temporary and is more painful for first-time mothers, women who have chosen not to breastfeed, and women who have delayed breastfeeding for 24 hours or more after delivery. If you begin feeding when you're engorged, you'll feel something akin to your arms being ripped out of their sockets; in other words, it HURTS! Request that your doctor recommend an appropriate pain killer to help under these circumstances. Another option is to request an oxytocin nasal spray, which will help with milk let down, and help to relieve engorgement faster.

If you're not breastfeeding, the engorgement will usually cease on its own within 12 to 24 hours, without lactation suppressants (the drug bromocriptine, which inhibits prolactin). Although lactation suppression is still available for women who want it, the FDA has recommended that bromocriptine not be used to suppress lactation in non-breastfeeding women. Your breast milk will "dry up" naturally unless your baby is suckling.

The Freedom of "Expression"

The worst thing you can do when your breasts are engorged is to feed on a set schedule, such as every 4 hours for 20 minutes. These schedules are a thing of the past, and while many practitioners may still recommend a set schedule, lactation consultants maintain that you and your baby need to form your own "play it by milk" schedule. In fact, unlimited breastfeeding actually prevents engorgement. Meanwhile, not only will feeding on a set schedule lead to more engorgement, but your swollen nipples can become cracked and irritated as well.

To relieve the engorgement, you'll need to express the milk as often as you can. This means you should nurse as often as possible and as long as possible. (AOAP and ALAP.) In short: as much as the baby wants for as long as it wants. A typical pattern may go something like this: nursing the baby on one side, then taking "time out" for burping and a diaper change. Then, switching to the other side, and taking time out for a burp and diaper change. At the next feeding, you should try to reverse the order and offer the last-used breast first. Whether your baby prefers smaller "meals" or an "all you can eat" buffet, there's generally no right or wrong as long as your baby appears to be feeding until satisfied. Lactation consultants also maintain that limiting feeding time solely to prevent cracked nipples is absolutely not necessary. The only thing that will help your nipples is making sure your positioning is correct so the baby can get a proper latch. (See above for feeding instructions.) You should also resist the urge to skip your feedings or procrastinate feeding. If you do, more engorgement will be the result. The only way to relieve your breasts is to feed. Other suggestions for engorgement relief include

- Expressing milk via a breast pump prior to feeding. This will help your baby grasp the nipple better during feeding and can also help to build up a milk "freezer stash" for later. If this is difficult, a warm shower will help with milk let down.
- Soothe yourself with whatever works. Whether it's ice packs, warm towels, or hot baths or showers, do it. Chilling big cabbage leaves and wearing them inside your bra is reportedly helpful.
- Give your breasts and nipples some air! When you're finished nursing, or when you're not concerned about leaking, you should air out your breasts by leaving your nursing bra undone or going braless. Letting the nipples breathe will help to heal them if they're sore or cracked. Air and light are important features in nipple training.
- Avoid nipple creams. Don't fall for Madison Avenue nipple cream concoctions. Nipple care involves plain water and no soap. Your own milk is the best lubricating and anti-infective "cream" there is. Just rub a little milk on the nipples after feeding.

More Than a Mouthful: Twin Feeding

Since most twins (or more) are born prematurely, breastfeeding is essential to help get your babies' weights and energies up. Like any new mother who breastfeeds, you must also follow the ASAP rule. If your babies are staying in a neonatal care unit and you are unable to take them to your breast, express your breasts with a pump and have them fed with your colostrum.

The obvious question is: Will you have enough milk? Yes. Remember, your breasts work on sheer supply and demand. The more suckling, the more milk production. The problem with feeding two mouths is that you may never get relief from feeding unless you design a workable schedule. In addition, because your positioning is trickier to coordinate, you, of all mothers, should have a lactation consultant visit you within the first two days of delivery (i.e., before engorgement) or before birth.

You'll most likely begin feeding one twin at a time, then slowly graduate to the double "football hold" (the legs of each baby are backward under your arm while you cradle a head in each hand). And, unless you want to be a professional milk cow for the next few months, you must also invest in a breast pump and accept help from your partner, other family members, friends and so on, to bottle-feed your babies with expressed breast milk. It should also be stressed that often breast pumps are more trouble and aggravation than just breastfeeding on demand. In this case, your partner should help with house chores and leave the breastfeeding to you. If you do use a breast pump, the most effective are the electric rental pumps, with a double setup. The best manual pumps are the cylinder-type. The old "bicycle horn" pumps are bad news and should be banned. You and a lactation consultant can coordinate an agreeable feeding schedule that combines breast and bottle, which suits you and your babies. Accepting help also means that you shouldn't attempt to be a superwoman and worry about a messy kitchen or bathroom. Let your partner clean up, and share more in the usual household chores.

Breast Milk Ingredients

Like any food producer, you need to keep up your quality control. You are what your baby eats! If you haven't consulted with a nutritionist yet, now is the time to do it. You need to eat properly in order to make high-quality breast milk. This not only means eating the right foods, but eating enough food! Although you may be tempted to go on a weight loss program, don't! Weight loss will affect your milk supply. In addition, your body will instinctively tap into your "baby fat" (your pregnancy weight) and use it as fuel for milk production.

Traditional caloric thinking was that breastfeeding mothers needed to take in 500 additional calories per baby per day. So, one baby = 500 extra calories; 2 babies = 1000; 3 babies = 1500, and so on. These extra 500 calories are 500 calories above your prepregnancy calorie intake! Now research suggests that the "500 calorie per baby per day" rule may be too high. So the best advice, according to LCs is this: "Eat when you're hungry and eat good stuff!"

Garlic lovers and chocoholics beware! Strong flavors and spices will affect your breast milk and may not agree with your baby. Classic newborn irritants are: garlic, onion, cabbage (which cause gas), excessive dairy products (causing colic), and chocolate. You'll have to test and see. Many women find, for example, that after a Chinese/Szechwan pig-out session, their baby's digestive system reacts negatively to their milk. If, however, your baby doesn't mind your spices and choices, there's no reason to cut them out. All of the dietary "don'ts and nevers" discussed in chapter 3 apply here as well. Whether it's your placenta or your breast, your baby is still affected by what you're eating, drinking, smoking, and inhaling. So, better safe than sorry.

In the 1990s, nutritionists may not be as necessary to breastfeeding mothers as environmentalists are. You'll want to make sure that your fruits and veggies are washed to help eliminate pesticides, and you may want to rethink eating that trout from your brother-in-law's fishing trip. Any fish or seafood bought from a large grocery store chain is inspected and hence considered safe. Also be sure to read labels. Obviously, less processed food and more natural foods are better. In addition, why not contact an environmental association and find out where to buy the safest food and what to avoid? Investigate whether there are any nuclear or chemical plants in your area. Breathing contaminated air, drinking contaminated water, and eating pesticide-free food from contaminated soil will introduce contaminants into your breast milk. Make sure you know what you're eating and breathing.

A word about baby's burps and stools...

Don't be alarmed if your baby doesn't burp as much as you think he or she should. Breastfed babies swallow far less air than bottle-fed babies. Nevertheless, go through the motions of burping the baby after each side until she or he burps. Some babies need to lie down for a minute and then be burped. At first, newborns pass thick, black, tarry meconium stools. As the colostrum works its way into the system, the black tar yields to mustard and greenish colors.

Greenish black, greenish brown, brownish yellow, or just plain yellow are all normal shades of stools for your baby during the first few days of breastfeeding. If the green/mustard color persists after a week or so, consult your pediatrician. This may be sign of diarrhea. You should notice stools after every feeding (6–10 times a day). Frequency diminishes as the baby gets older. This frequency really varies from several movements per day to once a week. The more infrequent the bowel movements are, the larger the stools should be. If stools are small and infrequent, the baby may not be getting enough milk and you should consult an LC and pediatrician. How can you tell if your baby is getting enough? The baby who "pees, poos, and grows" is doing just fine!

The Breastfeeding Decision

There are numerous benefits to breastfeeding: It's more nutritious; it's cheap; it's convenient and safe; it's instant, fast food; it's available for as long as you need it; it helps your uterus shrink; it helps you lose weight; it helps you bond; and it can be done by working mothers with the aid of breast pumps. One Canadian study found that more mothers are breastfeeding now than at any time in the last 30 years. In 1963, 38% of all mothers breastfed; today 83% do it. It was also found that mothers over 36 were more adamant about breastfeeding than mothers under 30.

It's estimated that prior to delivery, 80–90% of all pregnant women want to breastfeed. After delivery, unless there's emotional support and adequate training and information about how to breastfeed, some of these women will just give up. According to public health nurses and lactation consultants, one of the most influential forces in the breastfeeding decision is your own mother. "I bottle-fed all of my children and you turned out just fine!" is a classic gibe. "Trust me, once you start, you'll be chained to the house. What about your husband and your career?" All of these little jabs can affect your decision. Well, don't let them. Women who bottlefed in the past often feel guilty about having not breastfed. Hindsight is 20/20. We simply know more today about what's "best for baby" than we did 30 and even 20 years ago. So if you want to breastfeed but are being discouraged by older family matriarchs, keep in mind that it is an undisputed medical fact that "breast is best" for baby physically and emotionally. There are some women who should not breastfeed, however. Bottle may be best if you:

- are HIV positive (never!)
- have hepatitis B or another active infection or virus that passes into breast milk (you still may be able to, but ask your doctor);
- are on any medication that passes into breast milk (often, you can substitute medications that *are* safe for breastfeeding—ask);
- have silicone breast implants that are 10 years old (In this case, you many still be able to, but discuss the risks with your doctor—see below);
- do not have enough glandular tissue in your breast, which can be due to damaged nerve endings from a previous surgery. (Even in this case, lactagogues can be prescribed);
- have babies with PKU or galactosemia;
- find it physically impossible to endure the pain of feeding (when nursing hurts, there is a reason: a bad latch or an INFECTION, discussed below); or
- have a baby with a cleft lip or palate. (These children can breastfeed beautifully with the right technique and/or aids. Check with a lactation consultant or contact La Leche League.)

Feeding Frenzies

Unfortunately, there are numerous myths regarding breastfeeding that have more to do with gossip than with breastfeeding. Below are eight common myths of the mid-1990s:

Myth: You know, if you have your baby when you're past 35, your breast milk isn't as nutritious as under-35 milk!

Fact: Having a first child late in life will not affect your breast milk at all. You'll be able to produce just as good milk at 40 as you will at 20.

Myth: You can't get pregnant while you're breastfeeding.

Fact: Breastfeeding has been touted as being a natural contraceptive. This isn't true. It has some contraceptive effect in the first three or four months, but it's not 100%. You'll need to practice a barrier method or use condoms unless you don't care whether you get pregnant so soon after delivery. Review chapter 8 for safe contraceptive methods in the postpartum period.

Myth: You have to stop breastfeeding if you're going back to work.

Fact: Nonsense! If you're going back to work, you can pump your breasts every three or four hours, freeze or refrigerate the milk, or use it for the next day's supply. This works well as a "milk supply" if you have a nanny or your child is in day care.

Myth: There's nothing you can do about sore nipples when you're breastfeeding. You just have to live with it.

Fact: Wrong again! Air and using your own milk as an anti-infective agent can work wonders, as well as learning the proper feeding technique to begin with. But even in extreme cases, avoid rubber nipple shields. These will interfere with lactation and may confuse the baby. Under these circumstances, see a lactation consultant and check if your positioning is correct.

Myth: You can't breastfeed if you have inverted nipples.

Fact: For inverted nipples, you can draw the nipple out with a needleless 10 cubic-centimeter syringe with a plunger inserted into the "needle" end. You can also purchase a shell that you put over the nipple that squeezes it down and makes it more available to the suckling child, but this seems to create the same problems as nipple shields.

Myth: You can't breastfeed if you have breast cancer or were treated for breast cancer.

Fact: You can breastfeed out of a cancerous breast. Your child will not catch breast cancer, and the milk will be just as good and nutritious. However, if you're currently undergoing treatment such as chemotherapy, hormonal therapy, or radiation therapy, you cannot breastfeed.

Myth: Breastfeeding from breasts with silicon implants is perfectly safe and poses no risk to your child.

Fact: Halt! You can technically breastfeed out of breasts with implants. However, there have been reports of health problems in children who were fed from breasts with implants. Worse, women with older implants are reporting alarming health problems, something that should make you question breastfeeding. The American College of Allergy and Immunology, based in Illinois, recently announced that breast implants tend to ooze and rupture with age. When this happens, women are at risk for silicone-associated disorders, which cause chronic fatigue, pain, hair loss, and a variety of other ill-health symptoms. In one study, out of 51 women with breast implants who complained of muscle and joint aches and excessive fatigue, the implants had ruptured in over half of them, and all of the women had their breast implants in for at least 10 years. Researchers have concluded that silicone in breast implants gradually oozes out to the outside surface of the implant. In some women, the body thinks that the silicone is a harmful foreign substance and launches an immune system attack on it. When the immune system does attack, the symptoms outlined above can develop. Do some research before you decide to breastfeed with implants! The silicon connection hasn't yet been scientifically proven, so discuss the situation with your breast surgeon or LC.

Myth: Bottle-fed babies don't bond with their mothers, which is why it's imperative to breastfeed.

Fact: Bonding has more to do with loving, holding, and nurturing your baby and providing it with a loving environment. If you're unable to breastfeed, or it is medically inadvisable, then don't feel guilty. Nobody can do more than their best. But if you can breastfeed but chose not to, you should be aware that you are opting to deny your baby the undisputed medical benefits of breastmilk. In other words, making an informed decision is crucial! As for sharing feedings, both breastfeeding and bottlefeeding moms can do this.

The Benefits of Breastfeeding

Your baby is a human being, not a calf. Therefore, a human baby is, of course, going to benefit more from human breast milk! Your breast milk is tailor-made for your baby and has at least a hundred ingredients not found in formula. In addition, your breast milk changes continuously to meet the needs of your baby. For example, the milk changes during a feeding, producing what's called a "hind milk" that contains more fat, giving the baby a sense of fullness and satisfaction. In climate changes, the milk adapts amazingly well, containing more water in hot weather and more calories in cold weather to keep up the baby's energy. During your baby's growth spurts, breast milk will also provide more proteins, fats, and calories.

Your baby can also digest breast milk more easily because it contains less sodium and protein, which puts less stress on your baby's kidneys. It also allows the baby to absorb calcium and increases protection against allergy, constipation, diarrhea, diaper rash, and general infections and viruses. Interestingly, breastfed babies also smell sweeter than bottle-fed babies.

It's been found that breastfed babies are generally less obese later in life (some studies estimate that bottle-fed babies are four times more likely to become obese), because breastfed babies stop feeding when they're full, while bottle-fed babies are urged to overstuff themselves. There is also lower cholesterol in breastfed babies, better mouth development, and fewer orthodontic problems. Evidence from several studies shows that women who breastfeed may significantly reduce their risk of breast cancer, ovarian cancer, and osteoporosis.

The World Health Organization now recommends that breastfeeding be continued until at least 2 years of age. This translates into breast milk only for the first 4–6 months of age, then breast milk mixed with solid foods until a year of age, then breast milk as a supplement until 2 years of age. One study tracked breastfeeding in 46 primitive cultures and found truly startling results: Tribes that weaned their infants at around 6 months had warlike cultures, while tribes that weaned between 18 and 36 months had peaceful cultures.

Finally, you can also share the breastfeeding with other family members by expressing your milk via a breast pump and storing the milk. Breast milk can be safely stored in the fridge for 48 hours and can be kept frozen for up to 2 weeks. In a separate door freezer, you can freeze the milk for up to 3 months. When you thaw the milk, do not microwave it; this will destroy some of the nutrients. Nor should you re-freeze previously frozen milk.

The Benefits of Bottle-feeding

Unfortunately, there are no unique physical or emotional benefits for the baby who is bottle-fed, but there are some valid benefits for you, which may translate into better quality care for your baby. For example, on the physical side, you are less likely to develop breast infections, while you don't have to worry about any medications passing into your breast milk. Emotionally, you may have more freedom with feedings since other family members can participate, but you will need to warm the milk and be concerned about temperature, something you don't need to do when you're breastfeeding. Other benefits of bottle-feeding is that your love-making will not be interrupted by common breastfeeding problems, and you can go on hormonal contraceptives sooner. (Note: If you're breastfeeding, making love after a feeding is always best to prevent let down during orgasm.)

What If I Don't Breastfeed?

The reasons listed earlier that may prevent you from breastfeeding incorporate a long list of conditions. So if you must bottle-feed for any of the reasons listed above don't feel guilty. Obviously, formula is better than potentially harmful breast milk. Formula is also not harmful in any way; it simply isn't as good as the real thing. Because of this, some would interpret a lack of breastmilk as "harmful," but it's more akin to the difference between canned vegetables and fresh. An excellent solution is to search for donated breast milk from a friend, family member, or third person your doctor/midwife can recommend. Obviously, it's important that your donor is someone you know or trust so that her breast milk isn't suspect (carrying HIV, for example).

As for the emotional bonding issue: to date, psychiatrists report no significant differences between breastfed and bottlefed children. In fact, the only thing that is encouraged is quality bonding.

Common Breast Infections

Breasts and nipples are like any other part of the body: They can get infected too! Antibiotics will fix this. The most common infection is called lactational mastitis, an inflammation of the breast due to bacteria trapped in milk. This happens during breastfeeding. Here, bacteria get inside the nipple The breast gets red, swollen, and inflamed. Ten percent of the time an abscess will form, which can be drained via a needle or a tiny incision made in the breast. Lactational mastitis is sometimes referred to as a clogged milk duct, even though the clog occurs because of this inflammation. Although clogged ducts can occur when you don't have mastitis, they are more often a symptom of it. About 10% of all first-time breastfeeders will develop lactational mastitis. Sometimes a fever and chills can accompany the infection, which is treated with simple antibiotics safe for breastfeeding. In fact, one LC told me that any nursing mother who thinks she has the flu, has mastitis until proven otherwise! It's crucial that you do not stop breastfeeding when you have mastitis because this can lead to an abscess.

There is also such a thing as nonlactational mastitis. This is a bacterial breast infection in nonlactating women. Bacteria get deeper inside the breast somehow. Diabetic women are prone to this for the same reasons they are for yeast infections. Here, the breast can develop skin boils, and you can also have flu-like symptoms. Antibiotics take care of this, too.

Chronic subareolar abscess is an infection of the sebaceous glands around the nipples. Bacteria are the culprit again and get inside the glands via breastfeeding or lovemaking suckling. The glands get blocked and your breasts get red and form painful boils. The gland needs to be surgically opened or the infection will keep coming back. Antibiotics and minor breast surgery are the treatments.

Your breast can also develop a milk cyst. This is absolutely nothing to worry about, but until you have the milk cyst diagnosed, you may have a bit of a scare. Essentially, you should perform a breast self-examination every month or so and look for any suspicious lumps or changes in your breast during feeding. A milk cyst is simply a self-contained lump in your breast filled with milk. Your doctor can easily aspirate the cyst with a fine, long needle.

Nipple Problems

Blocked nipples due to dried-up milk, a plugged or blocked duct, are a common breastfeeding problem that may make you suspect a larger infection. Before you panic, just clean your nipples with a moistened sterile cotton swab and see if your feeding problems dissipate. You can also try expressing the milk in a warm shower.

Again, nipples can get sore, dry, cracked, and itchy. This can be caused by nursing, rashes, dry skin, or even eczema (if you have eczema on other parts of your body, for example). Eczema will often occur when solids are introduced into the baby's diet. You're reacting to the solids in the baby's mouth. As mentioned earlier, cracked, sore nipples can be relieved with your own breast milk, and plenty of light and air. You should also rinse your bras with vinegar to eliminate any laundry soap residue. If a rash or dry skin persists, see your doctor. There is a rare kind of breast cancer, known as Paget's disease that is characterized by a rash or dryness around one nipple and very rarely around both.

In extreme cases of nipple irritation, Raynaud's syndrome can develop, where the nipple turns white and is extremely painful during and after feedings. The cure for this is correcting a bad latch and taking painkillers that are safe to use during breastfeeding. Consult your doctor or lactation consultant about appropriate pain relief.

Finally, yeast or bacteria can get into the nipple, causing impetigo (a bacterial infection) or thrush (a yeast infection). Either infection can cause symptoms of burning and irritation. Your doctor should culture your nipple to sort out what infection you have, and then either prescribe an antibiotic or antifungal.

Breast Self-Examination (BSE)

Every woman over 30 should be aware that she's living during a breast cancer epidemic. If you've never performed BSE before, get into the habit today. BSE is not about finding breast cancer; it's about getting to know your breasts. Whether you're breastfeeding or not, your pregnancy has brought about tremendous changes in your breasts. Unless you know what your breasts normally feel like and which lumps and bumps are just "you," you won't be able to recognize a suspicious breast lump.

BSE involves specific steps of feeling your breast at the same time each month. That way, you may be able distinguish suspicious lumps from milk cysts, enlarged lymph nodes, and so on. In addition, you can't know if a lump is suspicious and has remained unchanged unless you've been checking your breasts monthly. While ideally you should begin BSE by the age of 20, starting now, however old you are, is just fine. When you're breastfeeding, you should perform BSE on a monthly basis after feeding so your breasts aren't filled with milk. When your menstrual cycle returns, you'll need to do a BSE after your period ends, and if you're still feeding, after a feeding following your period. That way, your breasts are least tender and lumpy and you *won't* be mistaking PMS tenderness and lumpiness with suspicious ones. Make sure your doctor goes over the following steps with you:

1. Visually inspect your breasts. Stand in front of the mirror and look closely at your breasts. You're looking for dimpling, puckering (like an orange peel in appearance), or noticeable lumps (which you often can't see). Do you see any unusual discharge that dribbles out on its own, or any bleeding from the nipple? Are there dry patches on the nipple (which may be Paget's disease)?

2. Visually inspect your breasts with your arms raised in front of the mirror, and look for the same things. Raising your arms smooths out the breast a little more to help make these changes more obvious.

3. Palpation (feeling your breast). Lie down on your bed with a pillow under your left shoulder and place your left hand under your head. With the flat part of the fingertips of your right hand, examine your left breast for a lump, using a gentle, circular motion. Imagine that the breast is a clock and make sure

you feel each "hour," as well as the nipple area and armpit area.

4. Repeat step 3, but reverse sides, examining your right breast with your left hand.

5. If you find a lump, note the size, shape, and how painless it is. A suspicious lump is usually painless, about ¼–½ inch in size, and remains unchanged from month to month. Get the lump looked at as soon as you can, or if you're comfortable doing so, wait for one month. If the lump changes in the next month by shrinking or becoming painful, it's not cancerous but should be looked at anyway. If the suspicious lump stays the same, definitely get it looked at as soon as possible. Breast cysts are common, the size varies and may be tender.

6. If discharge other than milk oozes out of your nipple on its own, or if blood comes out, see your doctor immediately. Don't wait. By the way, blood in breastmilk is not uncommon, and could be caused by a cracked nipple.

7. If your nipple is dry and patchy, see your doctor immediately. Don't wait.

For your information, 90% of all breast cancers are picked up by women themselves, either accidentally or through BSE. At all times of your life, particularly when you're breastfeeding, BSE should become a monthly ritual. As you wean, and your breast decreases in fullness, or perhaps prepares for yet another pregnancy, breast changes will mean that you need to constantly familiarize yourself with your breasts. Finally, please continue your BSE throughout all stages of your pregnancy. You can get breast cancer while you're pregnant.

The final chapter discusses one of the most mysterious postpartum conditions: maternal blues and postpartum depression. For the postpartum body, not only the breasts need to be expressed, so do the emotions.

10

Postpartum Depression

For the most part, this book has focused on all the physical changes you experience with pregnancy and childbirth. This final chapter, rather appropriately, discusses the emotional changes you'll be feeling after childbirth.

You might have heard of the infamous "postpartum blues," which is sometimes confused with *postpartum depression*. However, the phrase "postpartum depression" has been used incorrectly by the media, confusing three separate psychiatric conditions that occur in the postpartum phase. This chapter is designed to give you the facts about depression, psychosis, and maternal blues, and also provides information about a common postpartum thyroid condition that is often misdiagnosed as postpartum depression.

What's Going On?

Documented mental disturbances following pregnancy have a long history. However, the connection between depression and pregnancy wasn't really studied until the 1960s. First, normal fatigue and feelings of "let-down" in that you've been excited and preparing for the birth, are common and normal. True postpartum psychological and emotional disturbances range from what's known as maternal blues to true postpartum depression, where one experiences symptoms of major depression or clinical depression (discussed below), to something known as postpartum psychosis, the kind of diagnosis made in a situation where a woman loses contact with reality. She may hear voices, have delusions, and in extreme cases, women have been known to kill their newborns, believing they were evil or abnormal in some way. Postpartum psychosis occurs in 2 out of every 1,000 deliveries and is not as uncommon as one is often led to believe.

Maternal Blues

Eighty percent of all women after delivery will suffer from maternal blues. The maternal blues are common, nothing to worry about, and transitory, meaning short-term. This condition usually occurs within the first 10 days (3 or 4 days on average) after delivery and usually lasts only for a couple of weeks.

Symptoms of the maternal blues are frequent crying episodes, feelings of sadness, low energy, anxiety, insomnia, restlessness, and irritability. These symptoms are seen in all classes and cultures, and there's no specific link between these symptoms and hormonal changes. Women who experience these feelings should feel comforted that they are normal and will pass.

What causes maternal blues?

Maternal blues are most likely caused by enormous hormonal shifts in your body. However, there isn't any real documented proof that what you're feeling is hormonal. Since we do know that hormonal shifts definitely cause premenstrual mood swings as well as menopausal mood swings, and we do know that estrogen levels are depleted after childbirth, it's likely that hormones are the culprits. Estrogen actually functions like a weak antidepressant.

Nevertheless, there are other causes that have to do with an enormous lifestyle shift. These include an increase in stress and responsibility, worry about your newborn, physical discomfort associated with the postpartum "physique," and possible exhaustion following labor and delivery.

There is also a kind of "let-down" that some women experience. During pregnancy you experience a lot of excitement and anticipation about the big day. Then, when the big day arrives, you experience an enormous physical strain, all of the energy and excitement you've invested in the experience needs an emotional outlet, and all the attention switches to the baby, so you cry. Similar feelings tend to follow weddings and big trips. In this case, though, one kind of adventure is over, but a new adventure is beginning.

New family conflicts often surface after delivery, too. If this is a first grandchild, the emotional tug-of-war between the two (or more) sets of grandparents may contribute to your stress. And don't forget—baby naming, baby naming ceremonies, christenings, baptisms, circumcision decisions, and *bris* planning take their toll on your stress levels, and can create dismal conflicts that are never settled. These family wars often interfere with you and your partner's relationship and enjoyment of the newborn.

If you're on maternity leave, your sudden change in daily activities may be a shock to your system, and you may have difficulty adjusting to your new schedule (or the horrors of daytime television). And, too often, babies are planned as a way to patch up relationship problems between partners. This is truly disastrous and usually creates more holes than patches.

What should you do?

Give it a couple of weeks and see if you feel any better. If these feelings persist, you should consult your doctor, or seek out counseling and explore whether your feelings are truly related to your postpartum condition or are perhaps related to other problems that are only now surfacing. Pregnancy can mask relationship problems that you may not have been aware of, or expose relationship problems. The pregnancy also masks lifestyle ruts that will eventually resurface after delivery. In other words, don't expect old problems to disappear just because you've had a baby.

Postpartum Depression (PPD)

Postpartum depression is more serious and persistent and affects 10–15% of the postpartum population. This depression can begin at any time after delivery, from the first few hours to a few weeks after the birth. These symptoms include a kind of apathetic mood, loss of interest in formerly pleasurably activities, change in appetite (usually decreased), fatigue, guilt, self-loathing, suicidal thoughts, and poor concentration and memory, and sleep disturbances (early awakening and unable to fall back asleep). When these feelings last for more than a couple of weeks, the consequences can be truly negative, leading to bonding problems and relationship trouble. However, women don't go from the maternal blues to depression. You can feel well after delivery and then suddenly develop postpartum depression.

Causes of PPD

The triggers of postpartum depression are now understood to be identical to those sited as causes for the milder maternal blues. But women at risk for this more serious depression are those with a family history of it and who are predisposed to chemical imbalances in the brain. Women who have a poor support system at home (spouseless, bad relationship with partner, teenage mothers, and so on) have higher levels of stress, which can change levels of hormones in the adrenal glands, and push them beyond the "blues" into a true biologic depression.

Interestingly, in some studies, a significant portion of new fathers suffer from postpartum stress and a form of the blues. This definitely suggests that the causes of the blues are not rooted exclusively in hormonal changes or brain chemistry changes but in lifestyle changes. This is particularly true in milder forms of depression.

Treating PPD

If you do begin to notice these feelings, treatment is available through your obstetrician, primary care physician, or a psychiatrist. You may just need counseling or you may need to be put on antidepressant medication. Counseling can vary from short-term "sorting out your life" chats to intense psychotherapy. It really depends on the severity of your symptoms. The best way to find a psychiatrist is through a referral from your doctor or midwife. Newer medications are available that are remarkably effective. For example, postpartum depression can often be treated in as short a time as two weeks with the right drugs and dosages.

There are now a number of postpartum support groups where you can talk to other women who are in the same boat. This may help you put all your feelings into a healthier perspective.

If you are taking medications for your condition, you may not be able to breastfeed. Some of the older antidepressants can be very harmful to your newborn if they get into the breastmilk. In addition, you should only agree to medication if it is clearly indicated. If your doctor recommends an antidepressant on your first visit, you should definitely find out why. Sometimes hormonal supplements are prescribed as well. In some instances, a therapist may suggest that you get some extra help at home until you're on your feet again.

Finally, about 10% of all women after pregnancy will develop a condition called postpartum thyroiditis, where the thyroid becomes inflamed after delivery and becomes either overactive or underactive. Unfortunately, many women who have postpartum thyroiditis are misdiagnosed as having postpartum depression. This is discussed further below. For these women, a diagnosis of postpartum depression can be enough to drive them crazy!

Postpartum Psychosis

This is the stuff of which TV movies are made. Postpartum psychosis can be very serious and can require hospitalization. This affects a very small portion of women and begins in the first month after delivery. Basically, you're totally out of touch with the world around you. HINT: If you're able to read this book, you don't have postpartum psychosis!

This condition usually indicates other psychiatric disorders, but women can suddenly develop the following psychotic symptoms: delusions that the child is dead or defective, denial that the birth ever took place, or hearing voices (inside their head) that tell them to harm the infant. Accompanying symptoms usually include the biological depressive problems such as sleep disorders, poor concentration, loss of energy, and hence, difficulty caring for the child. Women at risk are those with:

- a past history of a psychotic episode or a past diagnosis of postpartum psychosis;
- women who are bipolar manic-depressive or schizophrenic (normally controlled with medication);
- women who have had a cesarean section (this is an actual statistic, believe it or not, but don't take it too seriously); and
- women with a family history of psychosis.

Postpartum psychosis is a serious psychiatric illness that needs to be treated with medications, which usually work quite nicely. In some cases, the infant may need to be placed in foster care or in the home of another family member.

Postpartum Thyroiditis

The thyroid gland is responsible for making thyroid hormone, which drives the function of every cell in your body. If your gland is either overproducing or underproducing thyroid hormone, your energy levels and emotional responses will be greatly affected. A significant portion of all women diagnosed with postpartum depression are not depressed at all but are suffering from a thyroid condition common in the postpartum phase: postpartum thyroiditis (inflammation of the thyroid gland). This is often a short-lived condition that tends to clear up on its own a few weeks after delivery.

Postpartum thyroiditis is a recently discovered health problem that is beginning to change the way postpartum depression is perceived in the medical community. It occurs in roughly 10% of all women after delivery. This translates into a huge number of women who will be relieved to know that their feelings of depression have a physical cause. Moreover, this figure does not include those women who will develop a permanent thyroid problem during or after pregnancy, accounting for at least 5% of the overall female population. These more permanent thyroid diseases are discussed in chapter 2.

Why Does Postpartum Thyroiditis Occur?

During pregnancy, you're extremely vulnerable to autoimmune (self-attacking) diseases, such as diabetes and thyroid diseases, due to a pregnancy-induced immunodeficiency. If you manage to avoid an autoimmune disorder during pregnancy, after delivery your immune system sometimes rebounds into a "super-immunodeficient" state instead of its normal, prepregnancy "on the lookout" state. Some women who may be borderline thyroid disease sufferers are especially susceptible to thyroid trouble after delivery. Their immune systems hold out just long enough to escape the thyroid problem during the pregnancy. Then, when it's all over, the immune system "relaxes" slightly, takes a deep breath, and a mini-thyroid condition sneaks past it. In this case, the thyroid condition is usually a short-lived, temporary condition that causes inflammation of the thyroid gland.

When you have this condition, your body produces "attack" antibodies to your own thyroid gland. As a result, your thyroid tissue is damaged and leaks potent thyroid hormone into your bloodstream, creating a situation where you have too much thyroid hormone (known as hyperthyroidism). After that happens, your wounded thyroid gland isn't able to produce enough thyroid hormone later on and can malfunction, creating a thyroid hormone "drought" in your body (known as hypothyroidism).

Women who experience one bout of postpartum thyroiditis are destined to relive the experience with each subsequent pregnancy. Unfortunately, there's no way to prevent the condition, but there's a simple way to diagnose and treat it, discussed below.

Symptoms

Symptoms of postpartum thyroiditis come in two groups; the group of symptoms you suffer depends on whether you're hyperthyroid or hypothyroid. It's more common to suffer from hypothyroid symptoms than hyperthyroid symptoms, however.

If you're hyperthyroid...

Your body speeds up and becomes overworked. Normally, you'd notice several physical symptoms that might tip your doctor off to a thyroid problem, but after delivery your postpartum state masks these symptoms. For example, when you're hyperthyroid, your heart rate increases, but since your heart rate increases during pregnancy anyway, most postpartum women do not notice this classic symptom. Other physical symptoms are weight loss, excessive perspiration, an intolerance to heat, irregular periods (not relevant in your case), and diarrhea, all physical symptoms you might attribute to your postpartum condition.

What you will notice, however, are some or all of the emotional symptoms: exhaustion, insomnia, irritability, restlessness and nervousness, anxiety, and general fatigue (caused by the insomnia). Until recently, any postpartum woman exhibiting these emotional symptoms was told she was suffering from either maternal blues or, after the symptoms persisted, postpartum depression. Obviously, when these emotional symptoms are caused by a physical problem, no amount of psychotherapy will make you feel better, which may exacerbate the symptoms!

If you're hypothyroid...

Your body slows down, creating some classic physical symptoms that, again, are completely masked by your postpartum condition. These include: constipation, bloating and fluid retention, a decreased appetite, lack of sex drive, dry hair, dry skin, intolerance to cold temperatures, and irregular periods (totally irrelevant in your case). As you can see, virtually no postpartum woman would notice any of these physical symptoms.

What you *will* notice are emotional symptoms: extreme fatigue and lethargy, depression, and tiredness and sluggishness regardless of how much sleep you get. And guess what? All of these symptoms can easily be misdiagnosed as maternal blues at first and postpartum depression later.

Diagnosing Postpartum Thyroiditis

Today, it should be standard practice for all pregnant women in North America to have their thyroid glands tested after delivery if they're displaying symptoms of maternal blues, postpartum depression, or thyroid disease. Regardless of how you feel, request that your doctor perform a thyroid function test after you deliver preferably before you're discharged. This simple blood test will determine whether you're either over- or underproducing thyroid hormone. If your thyroid test is normal yet you still have symptoms of PPD or maternal blues, you can rule out a physical cause for your symptoms. End of story.

Treating Postpartum Thyroiditis

Most women will experience hypothyroid symptoms. In this case, you may be monitored and given no medication unless the symptoms are severe enough to warrant it. Medication is one, tiny thyroid replacement hormone pill that replaces or supplements the thyroid hormone your body naturally makes.

If your hyperthyroid symptoms are severe, you may be placed on an antithyroid drug known as propylthiouracil (PTU), medication that quiets down your thyroid until it corrects itself. Treatment for hyperthyroidism is discussed in chapter 2.

Regardless of whether you're given thyroid hormone or PTU, you can still breastfeed safely.

Two Good Questions About
Postpartum Thyroiditis

You'll be hearing more about thyroid disorders and postpartum thyroiditis in the years to come. In fact, I have a file folder filled with misinformation about women and thyroid disorders. Here are the two questions that all postpartum women should know the answers to:

Q. I was diagnosed with postpartum thyroiditis over six months ago, and my thyroid condition doesn't seem to be going away!

A. You probably don't have postpartum thyroiditis, but postpartum *thyroid disease*. All that means is that you have a permanent thyroid condition that has developed after delivery. Most permanent thyroid conditions take the form of either Graves' disease (causing hyperthyroidism) or Hashimoto's disease (causing hypothyroidism). Request a referral to an endocrinologist, a specialist who manages endocrine problems such as thyroid disease or diabetes. Review *The Thyroid Sourcebook* for more information on thyroid disease.

Q. I'm currently being treated for a postpartum thyroid condition, but I'm still suffering from extreme emotional symptoms that don't seem to be related.

A. Then they're probably not. Remember, just because you have postpartum thyroiditis or a permanent thyroid condition doesn't mean you can't also develop maternal blues, postpartum depression, or another more permanent psychiatric problem. In addition to seeing an endocrinologist, you should be under the care of a psychiatrist as well.

If you're like me, this may be the first paragraph you read. As I stated in the introduction, this book is designed to give you all the information you need about your pregnant and postpartum body. So while you won't find too much information on fetal development, child care, or the several neonatal conditions that can develop, you will find everything and I mean everything you need to know about managing your prenatal and postpartum health care, as well what to expect from the pregnant and postpartum physique.

In addition, there's lots of information for those of you who are in the high-risk category. Whether you're pregnant with twins, have diabetes or asthma, or are 40 years old and pregnant with your first child, you haven't been left out of this pregnancy sourcebook. Read it, share it with your friends, and don't be afraid to "get permission from the author" to photocopy certain sections. Good luck and good health.

Bibliography

10 Great Reasons to Breast-Feed. Pamphlet, Ministry of National Health and Welfare, Ministry of Supply and Services. Canada, 1990.

10 Valuable Tips for Successful Breastfeeding. Pamphlet, Ministry of National Health and Welfare, Ministry of Supply and Services, Canada, 1991.

Abrams, Barbara. "Prenatal Weight Gain and Postpartum Weight Retention: A Delicate Balance." *American Journal of Public Health,* 83 (August 1993).

Adams Hillard, Paula, M.D. "Coping With Morning Sickness." *Parents' Magazine,* 65 (August 1990).

Arsenault, Gillian, M.D., I.B.C.L.C., family practitioner and certified lactation consultant, interviewed 1994.

Arsenault, Gillian, M.D., I.B.C.L.C., "You Learn the Darnedest Things When You Have Kids Or, What I Have Learned About Breast-feeding." *BC Health and Disease Surveillance,* 2, no. 10, September 13, 1993.

Boston Women's Health Book Collective. *The New Our Bodies, Ourselves* (New York: Simon & Schuster, 1992).

"Breast Cancer: Pregnancy Advisable?" Nursing 89, June 1989.

"Breast Versus Bottle." *Flare Magazine,* November 1993.

Brennan, Barbara, M.D., F.R.C.S. (C). "Prenatal Testing: Remove Some of the Guesswork." *Expecting: A Pregnancy Guide* 44, no. 4, (Fall/Winter).

Carson, Sandra A., and John E. Buster. "Ectopic Pregnancy." *The New England Journal of Medicine,* 329 (October 14, 1993).

Carty, Elaine McEwan, R.N., M.S.N., C.N.M. "Resuming Intimacy: Couples Need to Express Their Love." *Best Wishes* 44, no. 3 (Fall/Winter).

Casiro, O., M.D., F.R.C.P.(C). "Fetal Alcohol Syndrome." *Expecting: A Pregnancy Guide* 45, no. 2 (Spring/Summer 1993).

"Causes of Prematurity Associated with Inadequate Diet." *FDA Consumer* 27 (July-August 1993).

Charlish, Anne, and Linda Hughey Holt, M.D. *Birth-Tech: Tests and Technology in Pregnancy and Birth* (New York: Facts on File, 1991).

Creasy, Robert K. "Preterm Birth Prevention: Where Are We?" *American Journal of Obstetrics and Gynecology* 168 (April 1993).

DeMarco, Carolyn, M.D. *Take Charge of Your Body: A Women's Guide to Health* (Winlaw, B.C., 1990).

"Depressive Symptoms After Miscarriage (Tips from Other Journals)." *American Family Physician* 45 (June 1992).

Drife, James Owen. "Tubal Pregnancy: Rising Incidence, Earlier Diagnosis, More Conservative Treatment." *British Medical Journal* 301 (November 10, 1990).

"Early Detection of Ectopic Pregnancy: Use of a Sensitive Urine Pregnancy Test and Transvaginal Ultrasonography." *Journal of the American Medical Association* 266 (November 13, 1991).

"Early Umbilical Cord Cysts Detected in First Trimester." *Medical World News* 33 (April 1992).

Eden, Robert D., Robert J. Sokol, Yoram Sorokin, Helen J. Cook, Gail Sheeran, and Lawrence Chik. "The Mammary Stimuation Test: A Predictor of Preterm Delivery?" *American Journal of Obstetrics and Gynecology* 164 (June 1991).

Eisenberg, Arlene, Heidi E. Murkoff, and Sandee E. Hathaway. *What to Expect When You're Expecting* (New York: Workman Publishing, 1991).

"Essential Hypertension: Don't Treat in Pregnancy?" *Patient Care* 25 (April 30, 1991).

"Exercise During Pregnancy." *American Family Physician* 42, no. 3.

Freed, Gary L., M.D., M.P.H. "Breastfeeding: Time to Teach What We

Preach." *Journal of the American Medical Association* 269, no. 2 (January 13, 1993).

Frinton, Vera, M.D. "Your Changing Body: The Postpartum Period." *Best Wishes* 44, no. 3 (Fall/Winter 1992) .

Gander, Rosemary. "Checklist For Mothers-To-Be." *Expecting: A Pregnancy Guide* 45, no. 2, (Spring/Summer 1993).

Gander, Rosemary. "Guidelines: For a Healthy Pregnancy." *Expecting: A Pregnancy Guide* 44, no. 4 (Fall/Winter 1992).

Green, Debra, and Joanne Malin. "When Reality Shatters Parents' Dreams." *Nursing 88* (February 1988).

Guthrie, Diana W., R.N., Ph.D., and Richard A. Guthrie, M.D. *The Diabetes Sourcebook.* (Los Angeles: Lowell House, 1993).

Hales, Dianne, and Robert K. Creasy, M.D., with the March of Dimes. *New Hope for Problem Pregnancies: Helping Babies Before They're Born* (New York: HarperCollins, 1992).

Hamblin, Gail, R.N. "Normal Discomforts: How to Cope." *Expecting: A Pregnancy Guide* 44, no. 4 (Fall/Winter 1992).

Hamilton, Emily, M.D., F.R.C.S. (C.). "What Pregnancy Means for You and Your Baby." Synphasic Patient Education Series, Syntex Inc.

Hanvey, Louise, B.N., M.H.A., "Delivery Decisions: Check Out Your Choices." *Expecting: A Pregnancy Guide* 44, no. 4 (Fall/Winter 1992).

Hardman, Nancy, L.R.N., and Lynn Jones, R.N., M.H.Sc. "The First Three Weeks: 20 Questions About Those First 20 Days." *Best Wishes* 45, no. 3 (Fall/Winter, 1993).

Hazes, J. M.W. "Pregnancy and its Effect on the Risk of Developing Rheumatoid Arthritis." *Annals of the Rheumatic Diseases* 50 (February 1991).

Herman, Barry, M.D., and Susan K. Perry. *The Twelve-Month Pregnancy* (Los Angeles: Lowell House, 1992).

"Influenza Virus and Schizophrenia." *American Family Physician* 44 (September 1991).

Johanson, Sue, R.N., sex consultant, interviewed 1994.

Kitzinger, Sheila. *The Complete Book of Pregnancy and Childbirth* (New York: Alfred A. Knopf, 1984).

Kramer, Matthew F., Albert J. Stunkard, Kathleen A. Marshall, Shortie McKinney, and Jane Liebschutz. "Breastfeeding Reduces Maternal Lower Body Fat." *Journal of the American Dietetic Association* 93 (April 1993).

Kuboniwa, Faith, R.N., B.N.Sc. "Vaginal Birth After a Cesarean Section." *Expecting: A Pregnancy Guide,* 45, no. 2 (Spring/Summer 1993).

Kupfer, Andrew. "New Images of Babies Before Birth." *Fortune* 128. (August 9, 1993).

Lakusiak, Ellen. "Nutrition Matters." *Expecting: A Pregnancy Guide* 44, no. 4 (Fall/Winter 1992).

Lander, Debra, M.D., F.R.C.P. (C.), psychiatrist, interviewed 1993.

Lauersen, Niels, M.D., PhD. *It's Your Pregnancy.* (New York: Simon and Schuster, 1987).

Leppert, Phyllis. "The First Trimester—Weeks 0–12"; "The Second Trimester—Weeks 13–27"; The Third Trimester—Weeks 28-40"; In *The Columbia University College of Physicians and Surgeons Complete Home Medical Guide,* 2nd edition (New York: Columbia University Press).

Levy, Nancy. "Labor and Birth Guide." *Expecting: A Pregnancy Guide* 44, no. 4 (Fall/Winter 1992).

Love, Susan, M.D., with Karen Lindsey. *Dr. Susan Love's Breast Book* (New York: 1991, Addison-Wesley, 1991).

Marshall, Connie, R.N. *From Here to Maternity: A Guide for Pregnant Couples.* (Rocklin, Calif.: Prima Publishing, 1991).

"Maternal Weight Gain and Neonatal Outcomes (Tips From Other Journals)." *American Family Physician* 47 (February 15, 1993).

Lazar, Matthew, M.D., F.R.C.P. (C.), F.A.C.P., pediatrician/ neonatal specialist, interviewed 1994.

Mills, James L., Lewis B. Holmes, Jerome H. Aarons, Joe Leigh Simpson, Zane A. Brown, Lois G. Jovanovic-Peterson, Mary R. Conley, Barry I. Graubard, Robert H. Knopp, and Boyd E. Metzger. "Moderate Caffeine Use and the Risk of Spontaneous Abortion and Intrauterine Growth Retardation." *Journal of the American Medical Association* 269 (February 3, 1993).

Moore, Lori, M.D., F.R.C.P. (C), radiologist, interviewed 1994.

Morales, Karla, and Charles B. Inlander. *Take This Book to the Obstetrician With You* (New York: Addison-Wesley Publishing, 1991).

"Multivitamin Supplements and Morning Sickness (Vitamins and Minerals)." *Nutrition Research Newsletter* 11 (November/December 1992).

Noble, Elizabeth, with Leo Sorger, M.D., F.A.C.O.G. *Having Twins.* (Boston: Houghton Mifflin, 1991).

"One Out of 500 Miscarriages from Amniocentesis." *The Doctor's People Newsletter* 3 (October 1990).

Ory, Steven J. "New Options for Diagnosis and Treatment of Ectopic Pregnancy." *Journal of the American Medical Association* 267 (January 1992).

Policar, Michael M.D., F.A.C.O.G., vice president, medical affairs, Planned Parenthood Federation of America, interviewed 1993.

Peters, Dawn, R.N. "Grandmother-to-Grandmother: A Word About Breastfeeding." *Best Wishes* 44, no. 3 (Fall/Winter 1992).

Rosen, Keith. "Drug Use Associated With Preterm Birth, Low Birth Weight." *Alcoholism and Drug Abuse Week* 4 (August 5, 1992).

Rosenfeld, Jo Ann. "Bereavement and Grieving after Spontaneous Abortion." *American Family Physician* 43 (May 1991).

Rosenthal, M. Sara. *The Gynecological Sourcebook* (Los Angeles: Lowell House, 1994).

"Screening Recommendations for Gestational Diabetes Mellitus." *American Family Physician* 45 (January 1992).

"Significance of Bleeding During First Trimester (Tips From Other Journals)." *American Family Physician* 44 (November 1991).

Simkin, Penny, R.P.T.; Janet Whalley, R.N., B.Sc.N.; and Ann Keppler, R.N., M.N. *Pregnancy, Childbirth and the Newborn: The Complete Guide* (New York: Meadowbrook Press, 1991).

St. John Ambulance. *First Aid, Safety Oriented* (3d ed) (Ottawa, St. John Amblance, 1990).

Staseson, Sharon, R.N., B.Sc.N. "Post Partum Blues: What to Expect." *Best Wishes* 45, no. 3 (Fall/Winter 1993).

Sterken, Elizabeth. "Breastfeeding." *Expecting: A Pregnancy Guide* 45, no. 2 (Spring/Summer 1993).

Stevenson-Smith, Fay. "After the Birth (Recovering from Childbirth)." *Parents' Magazine* 68 (March 1993).

Swanson, Leila, "Talking About Twins." *Best Wishes* 45, no. 3 (Fall/Winter 1993).

"Tubal Pregnancies: Casualty of the Modern Lifestyle." *The Women's Letter* 4 (February 1991).

"Use of Ultrasonography to Diagnose Ectopic Pregnancy (Tips From Other Journals)." *American Family Physician* 42 (November 1990).

"Vitamin B_6 is Effective Therapy for Nausea and Vomiting of Pregnancy: A Randomized, Double-Blind Placebo-Controlled Study." *Journal of American Medical Association* 266 (November 20, 1991).

"Vitamin B_6 Therapy for Nausea in Pregnancy." *Nutrition Research Newsletter* 10 (July/August 1991)

Wald, Nicholas, Rossana Stone, H. S. Cuckle, J. G. Grudzinskas, Gad Barkai, Bruno Brambati, Borge Teisner, and Walter Fuhrmann. "First Trimester Concentrations of Pregnancy Associated Plasma Protein A and Placental Protein 14 in Down's Syndrome," *British Medical Journal* 305 (July 4, 1992).

Watson-MacDonell, Jo, R.N., B.Sc.N. "Episiotomy." *Expecting: A Pregnancy Guide* 44, no. 4 (Fall/Winter 1992).

Webb, Denise. "Eating Well." *New York Times* (November 3, 1993).

West, Karen, R.N. "Pregnancy's Progress." *Expecting: A Pregnancy Guide* 44, no. 4 (Fall/Winter 1992).

Wong, Kee-Lam, Fung-Yee Chan, and Chin-Peng Lee. "Outcome of Pregnancy in Patients with Systemic Lupus Erythematosus: A Prospective Study." *Archives of Internal Medicine* 151 (February 1991).

APPENDIX A

Where to Go
For More Information

Note: Because of the volatile nature of many health and/or non-profit organizations regarding funding and resources, some of these addresses and numbers may have changed since this list was compiled. I apologize for any inconvenience.

American Academy of Husband-
 Coached Childbirth
(AAHCC)
P.O. Box 5224
Sherman Oaks, CA 91413
818-788-6662

American College of Obstetricians and Gynecologists
409 12th Street SW
Washington, DC 20024
202-638-5577

American College of Nurse-
 Midwives
818 Connecticut Avenue NW,
 Suite 900
Washington, DC 20006
202-728-9860

American Foundation for Maternal and Child Health
439 East 51st Street, 4th Floor
New York, NY 10022
212-759-5510

American Gynecological and Obstetrical Society
c/o James R. Scott, M.D., OB-
 Gyn Dept., Room 2B200
University of Utah
50 North Medical Drive
Salt Lake City, UT 84132
801-581-5501

Childbirth Education Foundation
P.O. Box 5
Richboro, PA 18954-0005
215-357-2792

Childbirth Without Pain
Association
20134 Snowden
Detroit, MI 48235-1170
313-341-3816

Healthy Mothers, Healthy Babies
Coalition
409 12th Street SW, Room 309
Washington, DC 20024-2188
202-863-2458

Informed Homebirth
P.O. Box 3675
Ann Arbor MI 48106
313-662-6857

International Association of Parents and Professionals for Safe
Alternatives in Childbirth
(NAPSAC)
Route 1, Box 646
Marble Hill, MO 63764
314-238-2010

International Cesarean Awareness
Network
276 Clarks Summit, PA 18411
717-585-4226 (ICAN)

International Childbirth Education Associates (ICEA)
Box 20048
Minneapolis, MN 55420
612-854-8660

La Leche League International,
and Breastfeeding Reference
Library and Database
1400 N. Meacham Rd.
Schaumburg, IL 60173-4840
708-519-7730/Fax 708-519-0035

Maternity Centre Association
48 East 92nd Street
New York, NY 10128
212-369-7300

National Association of Childbearing Centres (NACC)
3123 Gottschall Road
Perkiomenville, PA 18074
215-234-8068

Positive Pregnancy and Parenting
Fitness
51 Saltrock Road
Baltic, CT 06330
203-822-8573

Read Natural Childbirth Foundation
P.O. Box 150956
San Rafael, CA 94915
415-456-8462

American Civil Liberties Union/
Reproductive Freedom Project
132 West 43rd Street
New York, NY 10036
212-944-9800

Planned Parenthood Federation of
America
(listed in your local phone book)

Attention: Canadians

The DES Cancer Network
DES Action USA
1615 Broadway
Oakland CA, 94612
510-465-4011

Special note to Canadians: The U.S. outperforms Canada in terms of organizations and resources. Although this list is peppered with Canadian resources, for any subject listed below, the best places to call are:

Toronto–Womens College
    Hospital
Regional Womens Health Centre
790 Bay Street, 8th Floor
Toronto, Ontario M5G 1N9
416-586-0211
(This is the best women's health center in the country.)

The Bay Centre For Birth Control
790 Bay Street, 8th Floor
Toronto, Ontario M5G1N9
416-351-3700
(Also provides counseling on abortion, adoption, prenatal care. Again, the best place in the country!)

Vancouver–Vancouver Women's
    Health Collective
175 West 8th Avenue, Suite 219
Vancouver, British Columbia
V5L 2Y7
604-736-5262

Montreal–Montreal Health Press
Box 1000
Station G
Montreal, Quebec H2W 2N1
514-282-1171

Nationwide—The Consumer Health Information Service, a joint project of the Faculty of Library and Information Science at the University of Toronto, Consumers Association of Canada, the Metropolitan Toronto Reference Library, The Toronto Hospital, and the Centre for Health Promotion, at University of Toronto, can be reached at:

789 Yonge Street
Toronto, Ontario, M4W 2G8
Outside Toronto: 1-800-667-1999
In Toronto: 416-393-7056,
    Fax 416-393-7181
All above numbers will put you in touch with the closest resource in your area. And all U.S. resources welcome Canadian calls!

APPENDIX B

Some Books that Might Interest You

This is a short list of titles I've compiled. All books below can be ordered from any bookstore if they are no longer on the shelves.
Note: For questions and recommendations about childbirth, pregnancy, parenting books, family planning, and other related topics, contact either:

Birth and Life Bookstore
P.O. Box 70625
Seattle, WA 98107
206-789-4444

Parentbooks
201 Harbord Street
Toronto, Ontario
M5S 1H6
416-537-8334
Fax: 416-537-9499

Aromatherapy for Mother and Baby: How Essential Oils Can Help You in Pregnancy and Early Motherhood. Allison England (1993, Vermillon, London).
Bestfeeding: Getting Breastfeeding Right for You. Mary Renfrew, Cloe Fisher, Suzanne Arms (1990, Celestial Arts, Berkeley, CA).
The Birth Partner: Everything You Need to Know to Help a Woman Through Childbirth (1989, Harvard Common Press, Boston).
Blooming Pregnant! Real Facts About Having a Baby. Cathy Hopkins and Kay Burley (1993, Robson Books).

The Breastfeeding Sourcebook. M. Sara Rosenthal (1995, Lowell House, Los Angeles).

The Complete Book of Pregnancy and Childbirth. Sheila Kitzinger (1989, Alfred A. Knopf, New York).

The Diabetes Sourcebook. Diana Guthrie, R.N. (1992, Lowell House, Los Angeles).

The Different Faces of Motherhood. Beverly Birns and Dale F. Hay (1988, Plenum Press, New York).

Dr. Susan Love's Breast Book. Susan Love, M.D., with Karen Lindsey (1991, Addison-Wesley, New York).

Expecting Change: The Emotional Journey Through Pregnancy. Ellen Sue Stern (1993, Bantam, New York).

The Experience of Breast Feeding. Sheila Kitzinger (1987, Penguin, New York).

First-Time Motherhood: Experiences from Teens to Forties. Ramona T. Mercer (1986, Springer Publishing, New York).

Giving Birth: The Great Adventure. Vernica McMahon (Janus, 1993).

Great Expectations and Inevitable Fears: Pregnancy and Birth. Kate Mosse (1993, Virago Press, London).

Mamatoto: A Celebration Of Birth. The Body Shop (1991, Virago Press, London).

The Midwife Challenge. Sheila Kitzinger, ed. (1991, Pandora Press, Hammersmith, London).

Miscarriage: Women Sharing From the Heart. Marie Allen (1993, Wiley & Sons, New York).

Mothering the New Mother: A Postpartum Resource Guide. Sally Placksin (1993, Newmarket Press, New York).

The Mother Zone. Marni Jackson (1991, MacFarlane, Walter and Ross).

No More Morning Sickness: A Survival Guide for the Pregnant Woman. Miriam Erik (1993, Plume, New York).

The Nursing Mothers Companion. Kathleen Huggins (1990, Harvard Common Press, Boston).

Parents at Risk. Ramona T. Mercer (1990, Springer Publishing, New Yor)

Postponing Parenthood: The Effect of Age on Reproductive Potential. Gale A. Sloan (1993, Insight Books, New York).

Pregnancy and Parenting. Phylliss Noerager Stern, ed. (1989, Hemisphere Publishing, New York).

Pregnancy, Childbirth and the Newborn, 3rd Edition. Penny Simkin (1991, Meadowbrook Press, New York).

Preterm Birth: Causes, Prevention and Management, 2nd Edition. Anna-Riitta Fuchs (1993, McGraw-Hill Health Professions Division, New York).

Take This Book to the Obstetrician With You. Karla Morales and Charles B. Inblander (1991, Addison-Wesley, New York).

The Kidney and Hypertension in Pregnancy. Priscilla Kincaid-Smith (1993, Churchill Livinstone, New York).

The Tentative Pregnancy: How Amniocentesis Changes the Experieince of Motherhood. Barbara Katz Rothman (1993, Norton, New York).

The Thyroid Sourcebook. M. Sara Rosenthal (1994, Lowell House, Los Angeles).

What to Expect in the First Year. Arlene Eisenberg, Heide E. Murkoff, and Sandee E. Hathaway (1989, Workman Publishing, New York).

What to Expect When You're Expecting. Arlene Eisenberg, Heidi E. Murkoff, and Sandee E. Hathaway (1991, Workman Publishing, New York).

When Parents Become Partners. Carolyn Pape Cowan and Philip A. Cowan (HarperCollins 199?)

Wise Woman Herbal for the Childbearing Year. Susan S. Weed (1986, Ash Tree Publishing, Woodstock, NY).

Woman to Mother: A Transformation. Vangie Bergum (1989, Bergin and Garvey, Granby, MA)

Your Baby and Child From Birth to Age Five. Penelope Leach (1993, Alfred A. Knopf, New York).

Index